# Percutaneous Interventions in Women

*Guest Editors*

ANNAPOORNA S. KINI, MD
ROXANA MEHRAN, MD

# INTERVENTIONAL CARDIOLOGY CLINICS

www.interventional.theclinics.com

*Consulting Editors*
SAMIN K. SHARMA, MD
IGOR F. PALACIOS, MD

April 2012 • Volume 1 • Number 2

SAUNDERS an imprint of ELSEVIER, Inc.

**W.B. SAUNDERS COMPANY**
*A Division of Elsevier Inc.*

1600 John F. Kennedy Boulevard • Suite 1800 • Philadelphia, Pennsylvania 19103-2899

http://www.theclinics.com

**INTERVENTIONAL CARDIOLOGY CLINICS Volume 1, Number 2**
**April 2012 ISSN 2211-7458, ISBN-13: 978-1-4557-3882-3**

Editor: Barbara Cohen-Kligerman
Developmental Editor: Teia Stone

*Interventional Cardiology Clinics* (ISSN 2211-7458) is published quarterly by Elsevier Inc., 360 Park Avenue South, New York, NY 10010-1710. Months of issue are January, April, July, and October. Subscription prices are USD 177 per year for US individuals, USD 119 per year for US students, USD 265 per year for Canadian individuals, USD 129 per year for Canadian students, USD 265 per year for international individuals, and USD 136 per year for international students. To receive student/resident rate, orders must be accompanied by name of affiliated institution, date of term, and the *signature* of program/residency coordinator on institution letterhead. Orders will be billed at individual rate until proof of status is received. Foreign air speed delivery is included in all *Clinics* subscription prices. All prices are subject to change without notice. **POSTMASTER:** Send address changes to *Interventional Cardiology Clinics*, Elsevier Health Sciences Division, Subscription Customer Service, 3251 Riverport Lane, Maryland Heights, MO 63043. **Customer Service: Telephone: 1-800-654-2452** (U.S. and Canada); **1-314-447-8871** (outside U.S. and Canada). **Fax: 1-314-447-8029. E-mail: journalscustomerservice-usa@elsevier.com** (for print support); **journalsonlinesupport-usa@elsevier.com** (for online support).

*Reprints.* For copies of 100 or more of articles in this publication, please contact the Commercial Reprints Department, Elsevier Inc., 360 Park Avenue South, New York, NY 10010-1710. Tel.: 212-633-3812; Fax: 212-462-1935; E-mail: reprints@elsevier.com.

Printed and bound by CPI Group (UK) Ltd, Croydon, CR0 4YY

Transferred to Digital Print 2012

# Contributors

## CONSULTING EDITORS

**SAMIN K. SHARMA, MD, FSCAI, FACC**
Director of Clinical Cardiology; Director of
Cardiac Catheterization Laboratory, Mount
Sinai Medical Center, New York, New York

**IGOR F. PALACIOS, MD, FSCAI**
Director of Interventional Cardiology,
Cardiology Division, Heart Center,
Massachusetts General Hospital; Associate
Professor of Medicine, Harvard Medical
School, Boston, Massachusetts

## GUEST EDITORS

**ANNAPOORNA S. KINI, MD, MRCP, FACC**
Director, Cardiac Catheterization Lab; Director,
Interventional Cardiology Fellowship
Cardiovascular Institute, Mount Sinai Hospital;
Professor of Medicine (Cardiology), Mount
Sinai School of Medicine, New York, New York

**ROXANA MEHRAN, MD, FACC**
Professor of Medicine; Director of
Interventional Cardiovascular Research and
Clinical Trials, Zena and Michael A. Weiner
Cardiovascular Institute, Mount Sinai School
of Medicine, New York, New York

## AUTHORS

**USMAN BABER, MD, MS**
Assistant Professor of Medicine, Department
of Medicine, Mount Sinai School of Medicine,
New York, New York

**LOUISE COATS, MRCP, PhD**
Specialty Registrar in Cardiology,
Cardiothoracic Centre, Freeman Hospital,
Newcastle upon Tyne Hospitals, NHS
Foundation Trust, Newcastle upon Tyne,
United Kingdom

**JENNIFER CONROY, MD, MBE**
Cardiology Fellow, Department of Medicine,
Mount Sinai School of Medicine, New York,
New York

**CRISTINA GIANNINI, MD**
Cardiac Catheterization Laboratory,
Cardiothoracic and Vascular Department,
University of Pisa, Pisa, Italy

**CINDY L. GRINES, MD**
Cardiovascular Medicine, Detroit Medical
Center, DMC Cardiovascular Institute,

Wayne State University School of Medicine,
Detroit, Michigan

**PAUL A. GURBEL, MD**
Cardiac Catheterization Laboratory, Sinai
Center for Thrombosis Research, Baltimore,
Maryland

**ANNAPOORNA S. KINI, MD, MRCP, FACC**
Director, Cardiac Catheterization Lab; Director,
Interventional Cardiology Fellowship
Cardiovascular Institute, Mount Sinai Hospital;
Professor of Medicine (Cardiology),
Mount Sinai School of Medicine, New York,
New York

**VIJAY KUNADIAN, MBBS, MD, MRCP**
Senior Lecturer and Consultant Interventional
Cardiologist, Faculty of Medical Sciences,
Institute of Cellular Medicine, Newcastle
University; Cardiothoracic Centre, Freeman
Hospital, Newcastle upon Tyne Hospitals, NHS
Foundation Trust, Newcastle upon Tyne,
United Kingdom

**ALEXANDRA J. LANSKY, MD**
Associate Professor of Medicine; Director
Interventional Cardiology Research;
Co-Director Valve Program, Yale University
Medical Center, Yale University School of
Medicine, New Haven, Connecticut

**ROXANA MEHRAN, MD, FACC**
Professor of Medicine; Director of
Interventional Cardiovascular Research and
Clinical Trials, Zena and Michael A. Weiner
Cardiovascular Institute, Mount Sinai School
of Medicine, New York, New York

**MARIE CLAUDE MORICE, MD, FACC, FESC**
Institut Cardiovasculaire Paris Sud, Massy,
Paris, France

**ANOUSKA MOYNAGH, FRACP**
Department of Cardiology, King's Mill Hospital,
Sutton-In-Ashfield, Nottinghamshire, United
Kingdom; Institut Cardiovasculaire Paris Sud,
Massy, Paris, France

**NITISH NAIK, MD**
Associate Professor, Department of
Cardiology, All India Institute of Medical
Sciences, New Delhi, India

**MASATAKA NAKANO, MD**
CVPath Institute, Gaithersburg, Maryland

**ELIANO P. NAVARESE, MD**
Interventional Cardio-Angiology Unit,
GVM Care and Research, Cotignola,
Ravenna, Italy

**VIVIAN G. NG, MD**
Columbia University Medical Center,
New York, New York

**FUMIYUKI OTSUKA, MD, PhD**
CVPath Institute, Gaithersburg, Maryland

**A. SONIA PETRONIO, MD**
Head, Cardiac Catheterization Laboratory,
Cardiothoracic and Vascular Department,
University of Pisa, Pisa, Italy

**AMBUJ ROY, MD**
Associate Professor, Department of
Cardiology, All India Institute of Medical
Sciences, New Delhi, India

**LESLEE J. SHAW, PhD, FASNC, FACC, FAHA**
Professor of Medicine, Emory University
Clinical Cardiovascular Research Institute,
Emory University School of Medicine,
Atlanta, Georgia

**KIMBERLY A. SKELDING, MD, FACC, FAHA, FSCAI**
Associate, Interventional Cardiology; Director,
Cardiovascular Research; Director, Women's
Heart & Vascular Health, Department of
Cardiology, Geisinger Medical Center,
Danville, Pennsylvania

**RAMYA SMITHA SURYADEVARA, MD**
Cardiovascular Fellow, Department of
Cardiology, Geisinger Medical Center,
Danville, Pennsylvania

**MOLLY SZERLIP, MD**
Section of Cardiology; Section of
Cardiothoracic Surgery, University of Arizona,
Tucson, Arizona

**UDAYA S. TANTRY, PhD**
Cardiac Catheterization Laboratory, Sinai
Center for Thrombosis Research, Baltimore,
Maryland

**RENU VIRMANI, MD**
Medical Director, CVPath Institute,
Gaithersburg, Maryland

# Contents

The evaluation of women who are asymptomatic or presenting for evaluation of stable cardiac disease symptoms has been the focus of much research in the past decade. The rationale for this research has been that fatality rates for coronary heart disease remain higher for women than men. Detection of high-risk populations is a core component of targeted therapeutic risk reduction and is a valuable way to identify women who may benefit from early intervention that could result in improved clinical outcomes. This article discusses the evidence on assessment of women with and without suspected cardiac symptoms.

Cardiovascular disease (CAD) is the leading cause of death worldwide in both women and men. Although the prevalence of CAD is less in women, those women affected by CAD die more often than men. Women are underrepresented in cardiovascular studies, making it difficult to determine the outcomes of different revascularization strategies. This review summarizes the current data on gender outcomes for percutaneous coronary intervention and coronary bypass grafting.

Acute coronary syndromes and ST elevation myocardial infarction are a major cause of cardiovascular morbidity and mortality in women. However, emerging data now suggest that the poorer outcomes of women undergoing percutaneous intervention may have less to do with differing vascular biology between males and females or the technical challenges of their coronary anatomy, but more with risk factors, such as age and comorbidities. Nevertheless, females have clearly been underrepresented in clinical trials, and further efforts are now required to properly define effective ways to tackle the risk-factor burden and clinical outcomes in women presenting to the catheterization laboratory.

Drug-eluting stents have become one of the mainstays of percutaneous coronary artery revascularization. Since their introduction, there have been many developments in this technology including the optimization of the stent platform, novel polymer coatings, and antiproliferative drugs. Although cardiovascular disease is the leading cause of death in women, the prevalence of obstructive coronary artery disease is lower, and women comprise a minority of patients included in clinical trials assessing the performance of drug-eluting stents. This article reviews the advances in drug-eluting stent technology and the studies reporting outcomes in women after implantation of these stents.

Ischemic heart disease remains the leading cause of morbidity and mortality in both genders in developed countries. Many women underestimate the effect of coronary artery disease on their health and as a result, the female population tends to be under-investigated for symptoms, with less-aggressive treatment approaches, leading to perceived worse outcomes in this group. Many assumptions about women are from studies where the female population is under-represented and in trials that do not account for gender differences. This article discusses percutaneous coronary intervention in high-risk groups and whether such a gender difference exists.

Compared with medical therapy, percutaneous coronary intervention (PCI) is associated with higher bleeding rates and more vascular complications. Although the rate of complications is decreasing, female sex continues to be an independent risk factor. Radial access for PCI is as effective as femoral access but is associated with significantly fewer bleeding and vascular complications. Although women are at higher risk for bleeding and vascular complications than their male counterparts, the use of radial access has decreased the complications to a level in the which the difference becomes minimal. More quality improvement studies are needed to identify strategies for reducing complications in this high-risk population.

It has been more than 3 decades since the introduction of percutaneous transluminal coronary angioplasty for the treatment of coronary artery disease, and the introduction of bare metal stents and drug-eluting stents (DES) has significantly improved clinical outcomes by decreasing rates of acute vessel closure and restenosis. This article reviews pathologic findings from male and female patients who had received coronary stents for acute coronary syndrome and died suddenly with or without complications of stent implantation, at early (<30 days) and late (>30 days) time points after DES implantation.

The underlying pathophysiology of ischemic complications during acute coronary syndrome involves thrombus generation at sites of plaque rupture and endothelial erosion, in which platelet activation and aggregation play major roles. This review discusses whether there are intrinsic differences in thrombogenicity between genders. In trials of acute coronary syndromes with dual antiplatelet therapy strategies, women tend to experience more ischemic events. Controversy exists surrounding the protective role of estrogens in the premenopausal woman. In vitro studies support the attenuation of platelet function by estrogen. Sufficient data support the presence of gender differences in thrombogenicity to promote further investigation in this area.

# Interventional Cardiology Clinics

---

**READ THE CLINICS ONLINE!**
Access your subscription at:
**www.theclinics.com**

# Preface
# Coronary Artery Disease in Women: Shyly Bold?

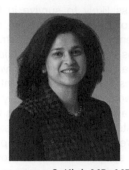
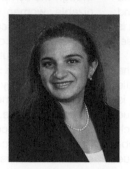

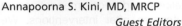

Annapoorna S. Kini, MD, MRCP        Roxana Mehran, MD
*Guest Editors*

*They must have perceived me as shy but they obviously didn't know what was going on in my heart.[a]*

Women are endowed to live longer than men. They demonstrate lower prevalence of coronary heart disease than men. They suffer fewer heart attacks than men and lag 15-20 years behind men for comparable incidence of acute events.

However, the risk factor profile is not as kind for women. Although dyslipidemia and cigarette smoking may be comparable to that of men, women show relatively higher prevalence of age-matched hypertension, diabetes, obesity, and lack of physical activity. The risk factors tend to cluster more often in women; the prevalence of two or more risk factors is more common than in men, and risk factor burden has increased significantly over the years. Although not too different in white women, the risk factors tend to be substantially higher for black and Hispanic women compared to men. The risk factors deteriorate considerably in postmenopausal years with worsening total and LDL cholesterol and small dense LDL; higher triglyceride; lower HDL cholesterol; decreased insulin secretion and increased resistance; visceral adiposity and poorer endothelial function; and elevated thrombogenic factors including fibrinogen, factor VII, and PAI-I.

Women, therefore, have a substantial lifetime risk of coronary heart disease, and more than 6 million women suffer from coronary disease in the United States alone. Cardiovascular disease prevalence among older people is higher in women than men, and each year since the mid-1980s more women than men have died from coronary artery disease. A substantially higher mortality rate has been reported in women after coronary artery bypass surgery. Similarly, primary percutaneous coronary interventions or even thrombolysis for acute coronary syndromes is associated with increased in-hospital mortality, and likelihood of procedural failure and complications.

Although the disease is neither adequately suspected nor optimally diagnosed in women, the outcomes are overtly different. Even the routine interventional procedures may not be as successful. We believe that the disease in itself is not the same as in men. Very recently, an association has been demonstrated between coronary artery disease preponderance in men and genetic make-up of the Y chromosome; 3233 biologically unrelated British men were genotypically characterized from the British Heart Foundation Family Heart Study, West of Scotland Coronary Prevention Study, and Cardiogenics Study cohorts. Of the 13 ancient lineages defined, carriers of haplogroup I (15% to 20% of the British male population) had about a 50% higher age-adjusted risk of coronary artery disease than did men with other Y chromosome lineages. The association was independent of traditional cardiovascular and socioeconomic

[a] With apology to Izabella Scorupco for modified adaptation of the original quote: "They remember me as this shy girl sitting under the table. But they obviously didn't know what was going on in my brain."

Intervent Cardiol Clin 1 (2012) ix–x
doi:10.1016/j.iccl.2012.03.001

interventional.theclinics.com

risk factors. These men showed downregulation of adaptive immunity as well as upregulation of inflammatory response pathways in macrophages compared with carriers of other Y haplotypes. These data show that predisposition to coronary artery disease in men might, at least in part, be determined by the paternal lineage of their Y chromosome and that this effect on risk of coronary artery disease is most likely mediated through the immune response, making the disease substrate different.

On the other hand, younger women, even in the absence of traditional hypercholesterolemia, die more frequently from plaque erosion. Smoking is the only established risk factor for underlying plaque erosion. This is in contrast to plaque rupture, which is the most important pathological substrate observed in men dying of coronary disease. Plaque ruptures are typically associated with classic risk factors including dyslipidemia. Erosive lesions are rich in smooth muscle cells with a paucity of macrophages, and most do not have an underlying necrotic core. Plaques prone to erosive lesions are rich in proteoglycans such as hyaluronan. Endothelial cells have lower potential for adherence to hyaluronan; endothelial cells in culture demonstrate decreased cell growth and increased propensity to apoptosis. Hyaluronan binds to CD44; CD44 receptors have been shown to mediate the adhesion of platelets to hyaluronan, and CD44 promotes atherosclerosis. The plaque erosion evokes more vasospasm and appears to be less atheromatous in nature. Erosive lesions are associated with increased frequency of distal embolization, more microvessel involvement, and increased myocardial necrosis. The microvascular differences probably account for increased mortality in women.

Coronary artery disease in women needs better scrutiny. The disease on the surface may be perceived as benign and presentation may appear to be shy, but the manifestation of the disease is bolder and complications are abundant. Even though the symptoms are milder and less recognizable, women are less likely to survive in the aftermath of acute coronary events than are men. Women consistently tend to demonstrate worse clinical outcomes in coronary interventions than do men. As such, a special issue of *Interventional Cardiology Clinics* on Percutaneous Interventions in Women seems justified and timely. In the current issue, a galaxy of authors discuss the similarities and contrasts in pathology of disease in women as compared to men, cryptic presentation of disease symptoms, interventional strategies, guidelines and recommendations in women, and outcomes after interventions. We sincerely hope that you enjoy reading this issue as much as the editors and authors have enjoyed developing it for you.

Annapoorna S. Kini, MD, MRCP
Mount Sinai School of Medicine
One Gustave L. Levy Place, Box 1030
New York, NY 10029-6574, USA

Roxana Mehran, MD
Mount Sinai School of Medicine
One Gustave L. Levy Place
New York, NY 10029, USA

E-mail addresses:
annapoorna.kini@mountsinai.org (A.S. Kini)
Roxana.mehran@mountsinai.org (R. Mehran)

# An Approach to Asymptomatic and Atypically or Typically Symptomatic Women with Cardiac Disease

Leslee J. Shaw, PhD

## KEYWORDS

• Cardiac disease • Women • Symptoms • Risk reduction

Much research in the past decade has focused on the evaluation of women who are either without cardiac disease symptoms or who are presenting for evaluation of stable symptoms. The prominent rationale for these clinical research efforts has been the report that the case fatality rates for coronary heart disease remain increased for women compared with men.[1] Moreover, this higher ratio of deaths for women compared with men has been reported since the mid-1980s.[1] Because detection of high-risk populations is a core component of targeted therapeutic risk reduction, it is a valuable approach for identifying women who may benefit from early intervention that could result in improved clinical outcomes. This article discusses the current evidence base on assessment of women with and without presenting suspected cardiac symptoms.

## RISK DETECTION IN ASYMPTOMATIC WOMEN
### Framingham Risk Score

For the asymptomatic woman, a recent clinical practice guideline synthesized the available evidence for the optimal strategy for assessment of risk in female patients. The integration of cardiac risk factors into a global risk score is the mainstay of cardiovascular risk assessment. The Framingham risk score (FRS) is one example of a global risk score that integrates traditional risk factors such as age, gender, blood pressure, diabetes, smoking, and cholesterol measurements. When the data from each of the risk factors are entered into a score, they produce an estimated 10-year risk of cardiovascular (CV) death or nonfatal myocardial infarction (MI). The scores are then categorized into low risk (<6% 10-year risk), intermediate risk (6%–20% 10-year risk), and high risk (>20% 10-year risk) of CV death or MI.[2] The FRS has been extensively tested in women and is currently supported by a class I recommendation in the recent American College of Cardiology (ACC)/American Heart Association (AHA) guidelines on assessment of CV risk in asymptomatic adults.[3] Following the calculation of risk, women with established heart disease who are classified as high risk are then targeted for therapeutic intervention and risk factor modification at secondary prevention levels.

### Family History of CV Disease

Family history of CV disease also has a class I recommendation. It is not included within the FRS, but an abundance of evidence exists that this risk factor is an important part of the clinical risk evaluation in women.

This recent guideline notes that the use of the FRS is most appropriate for asymptomatic individuals 40 years of age and older.

Emory University Clinical Cardiovascular Research Institute, Emory University School of Medicine, Room 529, 1462 Clifton Road North east, Atlanta, GA, USA
E-mail address: lshaw3@emory.edu

Intervent Cardiol Clin 1 (2012) 157–163
doi:10.1016/j.iccl.2012.02.001
2211-7458/12/$ – see front matter © 2012 Elsevier Inc. All rights reserved.

interventional.theclinics.com

## Reynolds Score

Major limitations of the FRS have been reported in women, including the underestimation of risk. The major driver of risk within the FRS is age, in which points are additive for older women. The underestimation of the FRS is most notably for women less than 70 years of age, for those outside the United States, and for women of diverse race/ethnicity.[3,4] In a recent analysis, 96% of women less than 60 years of age were classified as low risk by the FRS.[5] In practice, clinicians should consider other factors that are known to affect CV risk, including a family history of CV disease, the metabolic syndrome, obesity, and an increased high-sensitivity C-reactive protein. These factors have been integrated into a female-specific global risk score, called the Reynolds score.[6] Factors included in the Reynolds score include age, glycosylated hemoglobin (with diabetes), smoking, systolic blood pressure, total cholesterol, high-density lipoprotein cholesterol, high-sensitivity C-reactive protein, and parental history of MI at less than 60 years of age.[6] Use of the Reynolds score reclassified nearly 1 in 3 women with an intermediate FRS. Most of the women were reclassified into higher risk states. Thus, use of the Reynolds score improves detection of high-risk women.

## Second-Line Testing

For asymptomatic women, second-line testing is reasonable for those with an intermediate global risk score.[4] The recent ACC/AHA guideline provided a synopsis of this evidence, including the data on risk assessment with treadmill exercise and coronary artery calcium (CAC) scoring.[4] For exercise testing, the preponderance of evidence supports the usefulness of functional capacity and peak heart rate achieved as a prominent measure for risk stratification in women.[7–10] Nomograms have been devised that provide clinicians with age-predicted maximal exercise capacity and peak exercise heart rate measurements. Impairment in exercise capacity; notably that of 5 metabolic equivalents or less, is associated with higher risk status in asymptomatic women.[8,9] Moreover, a recent female-specific calculation of predicted maximal heart rate was published: 206−0.88(age in years). For asymptomatic women achieving less than 80% of predicted maximum heart rate, worsening survival has been reported.[7] Given the low prevalence of obstructive coronary artery disease (CAD) in asymptomatic women, exertional ST segment changes are not a good predictor of outcome; the exception is marked electrocardiographic changes.

CAC is another noninvasive testing modality that has an extensive evidence base for the ability to risk stratify women. The commonly used CAC score provides an estimate of the area of calcification on a computed tomography (CT) scan combined with the density of calcification.[11] A CAC score of 0 is low risk, 1 to 99 is mildly increased risk, 100 to 399 is moderate risk, 400 to 499 is high risk, and 1000 or more is very high risk.[12,13] Michos and colleagues[14] reported that most women with CAC significantly greater than the 75th percentile ranking for age had a low FRS, supporting the notion that subclinical atherosclerosis is prevalent in adult women. In a related report from the National Institutes of Health (National Heart, Lung, and Blood Institute Multi-Ethnic Study of Atherosclerosis), the prevalence of a high-risk CAC score of 300 or higher had an increased risk of CV death or MI.[15] Other reports have similarly reported effective risk stratification of women at high risk of CV events for those with a high-risk CAC score (ie, 300–400 or higher); including those of diverse ages.[16–18] In the recent ACC/AHA guideline, use of a CAC score is reasonable for women with an intermediate FRS; this has garnered a class IIa recommendation.

## EVALUATION OF SUSPECTED CARDIAC SYMPTOMS IN WOMEN

A synopsis of evidence on the diagnostic work-up of symptomatic women has been provided in a statement from the AHA.[19] Effective detection of CAD risk in women presenting with suspected CAD requires an understanding that accompanying chest pain symptoms need to be considered more broadly because of the greater frequency of atypical symptoms. Women have fewer exertional symptoms; more often with stomach or arm pain, dyspnea and associated anxiety, weakness, or fatigue. As a result, angina symptoms are less precise in the delineation of CAD risk in women.[20] For example, for a woman presenting with atypical angina, the probability of CAD varies by as much as 30%.[20] More recently, Cheng and colleagues[21] reported on the prevalence of obstructive CAD by coronary computed tomographic angiography (CCTA), a newly introduced noninvasive anatomic test. In this contemporary report of 5684 women, the prevalence of CAD increased with age but not with the typicality of symptoms (**Fig. 1**).[21] As such, these data support the indiscriminate nature of presenting symptoms in women, at least within the current knowledge base, and the importance of additional diagnostic testing to assess CAD risk for women.

There is an apparent gender paradox for CAD, in that women have less typical symptom presentation,

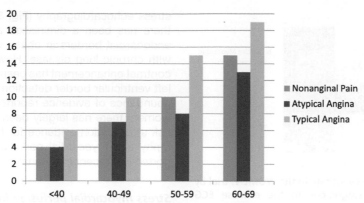

**Fig. 1.** Prevalence of CAD stenosis greater than or equal to 50% in women with suspected cardiac symptoms.

have a lower prevalence of CAD, but are older at the time of index evaluation, with greater degrees of co-morbidity and worse clinical outcomes.[22] This paradox can lead to a reduced intensity of clinical evaluation and less aggressive management of women.[23,24] From a recent report from Finland in 56,441 ambulatory women and 34,885 men aged 45 to 89 years, the presence of symptoms combined with demonstrable ischemia was associated with higher coronary mortality in women compared with men.[25] These findings support the notion that ischemia can provide important information to guide risk stratification of symptomatic women.

## Exercise Electrocardiogram

The exercise electrocardiogram (ECG) is commonly applied but reportedly has a limited diagnostic accuracy, with the ability to detect CAD in the setting of a positive test (ie, sensitivity) of approx-imately 60%. A similarly low accuracy has been re-ported to exclude CAD in the setting of a negative test (ie, specificity, ~65%). As with the asymp-tomatic woman, peak heart rate and functional capacity measures figure prominently in risk detection.[19] In one report, functional capacity was estimated with the simple Duke Activity Status Index (DASI), which provides estimates of metabolic equivalents and identifies women requiring referral to pharmacologic stress imaging.[26] Other limitations of exercise testing in women are noted in **Box 1**. For most women, the exercise ECG is bypassed for a more costly, imaging procedure, such as stress echocardiog-raphy or myocardial perfusion imaging.

## Stress Imaging

The critical question of when to refer a woman to a stress imaging modality was recently addressed in a randomized clinical trial enrolling 824 symp-tomatic women.[27] Women enrolled in the

WOMENs (What is the Optimal Method of Ischemia Evaluation in Women) trial were largely younger with a lower likelihood of CAD, including those able to exercise and achieve 5 or more metabolic equivalents of physical activity.[28] Women in this trial exercised to a median of 7 minutes on the modified Bruce protocol; as such, the results can largely be generalized to functionally capable women. Women were randomized to an exercise ECG versus an exercise myocardial perfusion single-photon emission computed tomography (SPECT) study and were followed for 2 years for the occurrence of major adverse CV events. At 2 years, the relative hazard for CV events was nonsig-nificant, with a hazard ratio of 1.3 (95% confidence intervals 0.5–3.5, $P = .59$) (**Fig. 2**). The implications from this trial are that, if a woman is capable of exercising, then the index procedure should be an exercise ECG. Women with intermediate or inde-terminate stress test results or those with high-risk findings should then undergo a stress imaging

---

**Box 1**
**Exercise ECG in women**

*Limitations*

- Exertional symptoms are of low predictive value
- Women have shorter exercise durations and are more likely not to reach maximal exercise
- Lower obstructive CAD prevalence
- Reduced diagnostic accuracy

*Strengths*

- A reported high accuracy in women with a negative exercise ECG in the setting of maximal exercise
- Good exercise tolerance portends excellent survival

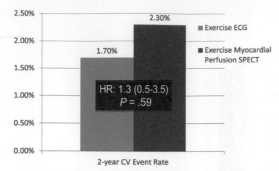

**Fig. 2.** Two-year CV event rate in the WOMENs trial by randomized test assignment to the exercise ECG versus exercise myocardial perfusion SPECT scan.

study. In the WOMENs trial, this was termed an ECG-first strategy to be followed by selective stress imaging in the setting of intermediate or high-risk findings. This trial also used the DASI as a means to identify women capable of exercise and, similarly to the Philips report,[26] could be used to differentiate women capable of exercise or for those requiring referral to pharmacologic stress imaging.

*Stress echocardiography*

Several additional stress imaging modalities are also worthy of mention because of their extensive literature base in female patient cohorts. Stress echocardiography provides delineation of rest and stress regional wall motion and function, with an extensive literature base for its diagnostic and prognostic accuracy.[19] Both exercise and dobutamine stress echocardiography have diagnostic sensitivity and specificity measures of greater than 80% in women.[19] Moreover, there are data for thousands of women on the ability of inducible wall motion abnormalities to differentiate risk.[29] From one report on 4234 women, the number of vascular territories effectively stratified risk in women undergoing exercise and dobutamine

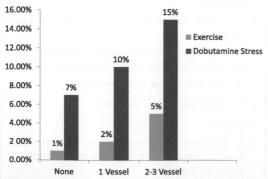

**Fig. 3.** Five-year CAD death rates in women undergoing exercise and pharmacologic stress echocardiography.

stress echocardiography (**Fig. 3**). In some cases, there has been a diminished ability to visualize endocardial borders in obese women and those with chronic lung disease. However, intravenous contrast enhancement has been shown to improve left ventricular border detection.[19] Because of the abundance of evidence reported in thousands of women, there has largely been a convergence of risk stratification evidence for both echocardiography and myocardial perfusion imaging, as reported in a recent meta-analysis.[30]

*Stress myocardial perfusion imaging*

For women undergoing stress myocardial perfusion imaging, the diagnostic sensitivity is high and ranges from 85% to 90%.[19] The diagnostic specificity is reduced because of breast tissue attenuation, but is commonly improved in the range of 80% to 90% with the integration of several factors including left ventricular function and wall motion assessment as well as the use of attenuation correction software or prone imaging.[19] Although there are numerous reports on the prognostic accuracy of stress myocardial perfusion imaging, one report in a large cohort of 6173 women and men reported a similar ability to risk stratify based on the segmental scoring of myocardial perfusion abnormalities on the stress SPECT examination.[31] For women with low-risk stress myocardial perfusion results, the annual CAD mortality is ~1% or less (**Fig. 4**). The risk of CAD mortality increases in a gradient manner with the extent and severity of stress myocardialperfusion abnormalities for both women and men. Reports have also validated these findings in ethnically and racially diverse patient cohorts.[32,33]

Stress myocardial perfusion imaging is associated with exposure to ionizing radiation. Thus, its use should be limited to women and men who are appropriate candidates for testing, based on the ACC appropriate use criteria.[34] Moreover, the primary radioisotope for evaluation of women

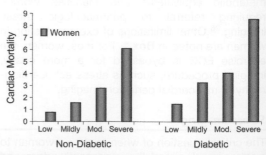

**Fig. 4.** Annual cardiac mortality in women undergoing pharmacologic stress myocardial perfusion SPECT.

should be rest-stress Tc-99m, unless imaging is required for viability purposes, with an average effective dose of ~12 mSv.[35] Because of a reduced exposure to ionizing radiation with Rb-82 positron emission tomography (at ~3 mSv), its use should be considered in women, although limited data are available regarding its accuracy in risk detection.

## CCTA

The final diagnostic testing modality to be covered in this article is CCTA. The evidence supporting CCTA as an effective diagnostic modality has grown considerably in the past 5 years, including evidence regarding its usefulness in women. CCTA is a noninvasive anatomic test with a high degree of spatial and temporal resolution as well as volume coverage. Significant attention to radiation dose reduction in the last few years has improved the overall safety profile of this modality. Currently, effective radiation doses are in the range of 5 to 8 mSv for most patients, with exception of obese patients.[36] There have been several controlled clinical trials that have reported a high diagnostic accuracy, with a pooled sensitivity of 94% and specificity of 80%. Both tests identify anatomic CAD and a reported strong correlation in findings is expected. More recently, there have been many findings on the prognostic accuracy of CCTA.[37–39] In one recent report,[37] the relative hazard for death was increased 2-fold to nearly 5-fold for women with multivessel CAD on CCTA (**Fig. 5**). Recent investigations of the value of non-obstructive atherosclerosis have shown promising preliminary findings that evidence of plaque may prove helpful in further identifying risk in symptomatic women with less than 50% stenosis.[38,39] In one recent report, nonobstructive plaque was associated with an increased mortality risk, beyond the extent of CAD, in women but not in men.[39] Further investigations are warranted to further delineate plaque composition as well as arterial remodeling and other adverse risk markers that may be visualized on CCTA.

## SUMMARY

This article highlights data on the effectiveness of screening in asymptomatic women and diagnostic testing in symptomatic women. In every case, articles that may be accessed for a more in-depth review on the subject are highlighted. The evidence on detection of risk in asymptomatic and symptomatic women is robust and can provide help in everyday clinical decision making. Evolving evidence and targeted treatment strategies that are optimized for women, including those with demonstrable atherosclerosis or ischemia with or without CAD, are being developed and will further aid clinicians in reducing the observed higher CV mortality in women in the United States and worldwide.

## REFERENCES

1. Roger VL, Go AS, Lloyd-Jones DM, et al. Heart disease and stroke statistics–2011 update: a report from the American Heart Association. Circulation 2011;123:e18–209.
2. Wilson PW, D'Agostino RB, Levy D, et al. Prediction of coronary heart disease using risk factor categories. Circulation 1998;97:1837–47.
3. Greenland P, Alpert JS, Beller GA, et al. 2010 ACCF/AHA guideline for assessment of cardiovascular risk in asymptomatic adults: a report of the American College of Cardiology Foundation/American Heart Association Task Force on Practice Guidelines. J Am Coll Cardiol 2010;56:e50–103.
4. Greenland P, Alpert JS, Beller GA, et al. 2010 ACCF/AHA guideline for assessment of cardiovascular risk in asymptomatic adults: executive summary: a report of the American College of Cardiology Foundation/American Heart Association Task Force on Practice Guidelines. Circulation 2010;122:2748–64.
5. Pasternak RC, Abrams J, Greenland P, et al. 34th Bethesda Conference: Task force #1–Identification of coronary heart disease risk: is there a detection gap? J Am Coll Cardiol 2003;41:1863–74.
6. Ridker PM, Buring JE, Rifai N, et al. Development and validation of improved algorithms for the assessment of global cardiovascular risk in women: the Reynolds Risk Score. JAMA 2007;297:611–9.
7. Gulati M, Shaw LJ, Thisted RA, et al. Heart rate response to exercise stress testing in asymptomatic women: the St. James Women Take Heart Project. Circulation 2010;122:130–7.
8. Gulati M, Pandey DK, Arnsdorf MF, et al. Exercise capacity and the risk of death in women: the St

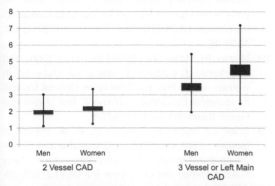

**Fig. 5.** The adjusted relative hazard for death from all causes for men and women undergoing CCTA with 2-vessel, 3-vessel, or left main CAD.

James Women Take Heart Project. Circulation 2003; 108:1554–9.

9. Gulati M, Black HR, Shaw LJ, et al. The prognostic value of a nomogram for exercise capacity in women. N Engl J Med 2005;353:468–75.

10. Mora S, Redberg RF, Cui Y, et al. Ability of exercise testing to predict cardiovascular and all-cause death in asymptomatic women: a 20-year follow-up of the Lipid Research Clinics Prevalence Study. JAMA 2003;290:1600–7.

11. Agatston AS, Janowitz WR, Hildner FJ, et al. Quantification of coronary artery calcium using ultrafast computed tomography. J Am Coll Cardiol 1990;15:827–32.

12. Shaw LJ, Raggi P, Schisterman E, et al. Prognostic value of cardiac risk factors and coronary artery calcium screening for all-cause mortality. Radiology 2003;228:826–33.

13. Budoff MJ, Shaw LJ, Liu ST, et al. Long-term prognosis associated with coronary calcification: observations from a registry of 25,253 patients. J Am Coll Cardiol 2007;49:1860–70.

14. Michos ED, Nasir K, Braunstein JB, et al. Framingham risk equation underestimates subclinical atherosclerosis risk in asymptomatic women. Atherosclerosis 2006;184:201–6.

15. Lakoski SG, Greenland P, Wong ND, et al. Coronary artery calcium scores and risk for cardiovascular events in women classified as "low risk" based on Framingham risk score: the Multi-Ethnic Study Of Atherosclerosis (MESA). Arch Intern Med 2007; 167:2437–42.

16. Raggi P, Shaw LJ, Berman DS, et al. Gender-based differences in the prognostic value of coronary calcification. J Womens Health (Larchmt) 2004;13: 273–83.

17. Bellasi A, Lacey C, Taylor AJ, et al. Comparison of prognostic usefulness of coronary artery calcium in men versus women (results from a meta- and pooled analysis estimating all-cause mortality and coronary heart disease death or myocardial infarction). Am J Cardiol 2007;100:409–14.

18. Raggi P, Gongora MC, Gopal A, et al. Coronary artery calcium to predict all-cause mortality in elderly men and women. J Am Coll Cardiol 2008; 52:17–23.

19. Mieres JH, Shaw LJ, Arai A, et al. Role of noninvasive testing in the clinical evaluation of women with suspected coronary artery disease: consensus statement from the Cardiac Imaging Committee, Council on Clinical Cardiology, and the Cardiovascular Imaging and Intervention Committee, Council on Cardiovascular Radiology and Intervention, American Heart Association. Circulation 2005;111: 682–96.

20. Diamond GA, Forrester JS. Analysis of probability as an aid in the clinical diagnosis of coronary-artery disease. N Engl J Med 1979;300:1350–8.

21. Cheng VY, Berman DS, Rozanski A, et al. Performance of the traditional age, sex, and angina typicality-based approach for estimating pretest probability of angiographically significant coronary artery disease in patients undergoing coronary computed tomographic angiography: results from the multinational coronary CT angiography evaluation for clinical outcomes: an international multicenter registry (CONFIRM). Circulation 2011;124: 2423–32, 1–8.

22. Shaw LJ, Bugiardini R, Merz CN. Women and ischemic heart disease: evolving knowledge. J Am Coll Cardiol 2009;54:1561–75.

23. Shaw LJ, Bairey Merz CN, Pepine CJ, et al. Insights from the NHLBI-sponsored Women's Ischemia Syndrome Evaluation (WISE) Study: Part I: gender differences in traditional and novel risk factors, symptom evaluation, and gender-optimized diagnostic strategies. J Am Coll Cardiol 2006;47:S4–20.

24. Bairey Merz CN, Shaw LJ, Reis SE, et al. Insights from the NHLBI-sponsored Women's Ischemia Syndrome Evaluation (WISE) Study: Part II: gender differences in presentation, diagnosis, and outcome with regard to gender-based pathophysiology of atherosclerosis and macrovascular and microvascular coronary disease. J Am Coll Cardiol 2006;47: S21–9.

25. Hemingway H, McCallum A, Shipley M, et al. Incidence and prognostic implications of stable angina pectoris among women and men. JAMA 2006;295: 1404–11.

26. Phillips L, Wang JW, Pfeffer B, et al. Clinical role of the Duke Activity Status Index in the selection of the optimal type of stress myocardial perfusion imaging study in patients with known or suspected ischemic heart disease. J Nucl Cardiol 2011;18: 1015–20.

27. Shaw LJ, Mieres JH, Hendel RH, et al. Comparative effectiveness of exercise electrocardiography with or without myocardial perfusion single photon emission computed tomography in women with suspected coronary artery disease: results from the What Is the Optimal Method for Ischemia Evaluation in Women (WOMEN) trial. Circulation 2011;124: 1239–49.

28. Mieres JH, Heller GV, Hendel RC, et al. Signs and symptoms of suspected myocardial ischemia in women: results from the What is the Optimal Method for Ischemia Evaluation in WomeN? Trial. J Womens Health (Larchmt) 2011;20:1261–8.

29. Shaw LJ, Vasey C, Sawada S, et al. Impact of gender on risk stratification by exercise and dobutamine stress echocardiography: long-term mortality in 4234 women and 6898 men. Eur Heart J 2005;26: 447–56.

30. Metz LD, Beattie M, Hom R, et al. The prognostic value of normal exercise myocardial perfusion

imaging and exercise echocardiography: a meta-analysis. J Am Coll Cardiol 2007;49:227–37.

31. Berman DS, Kang X, Hayes SW, et al. Adenosine myocardial perfusion single-photon emission computed tomography in women compared with men. Impact of diabetes mellitus on incremental prognostic value and effect on patient management. J Am Coll Cardiol 2003;41:1125–33.

32. Shaw LJ, Hendel RC, Cerquiera M, et al. Ethnic differences in the prognostic value of stress technetium-99m tetrofosmin gated single-photon emission computed tomography myocardial perfusion imaging. J Am Coll Cardiol 2005;45:1494–504.

33. Cerci MS, Cerci JJ, Cerci RJ, et al. Myocardial perfusion imaging is a strong predictor of death in women. JACC Cardiovasc Imaging 2011;4:880–8.

34. Hendel RC, Berman DS, Di Carli MF, et al. ACCF/ASNC/ACR/AHA/ASE/SCCT/SCMR/SNM 2009 Appropriate Use Criteria for Cardiac Radionuclide Imaging: a Report of the American College of Cardiology Foundation Appropriate Use Criteria Task Force, the American Society of Nuclear Cardiology, the American College of Radiology, the American Heart Association, the American Society of Echocardiography, the Society of Cardiovascular Computed Tomography, the Society for Cardiovascular Magnetic Resonance, and the Society of Nuclear Medicine. J Am Coll Cardiol 2009; 53:2201–29.

35. Cerqueira MD, Allman KC, Ficaro EP, et al. Recommendations for reducing radiation exposure in myocardial perfusion imaging. J Nucl Cardiol 2010;17:709–18.

36. Halliburton SS, Abbara S, Chen MY, et al. SCCT guidelines on radiation dose and dose-optimization strategies in cardiovascular CT. J Cardiovasc Comput Tomogr 2011;5:198–224.

37. Min JK, Dunning A, Lin FY, et al. Age- and sex-related differences in all-cause mortality risk based on coronary computed tomography angiography findings results from the International Multicenter CONFIRM (Coronary CT Angiography Evaluation for Clinical Outcomes: an International Multicenter Registry) of 23,854 patients without known coronary artery disease. J Am Coll Cardiol 2011;58: 849–60.

38. Lin FY, Shaw LJ, Dunning AM, et al. Mortality risk in symptomatic patients with nonobstructive coronary artery disease: a prospective 2-center study of 2,583 patients undergoing 64-detector row coronary computed tomographic angiography. J Am Coll Cardiol 2011;58:510 9.

39. Shaw LJ, Min JK, Narula J, et al. Sex differences in mortality associated with computed tomographic angiographic measurements of obstructive and nonobstructive coronary artery disease: an exploratory analysis. Circ Cardiovasc Imaging 2010;3:473–81.

# Revascularization Strategies in Women with Stable Cardiovascular Disease: What do the Trials Reveal?

Molly Szerlip, MD[a], Cindy L. Grines, MD[b],*

## KEYWORDS

- Coronary revascularization • Gender outcomes
- Coronary artery disease
- Percutaneous coronary revascularization
- Coronary artery bypass grafting

Cardiovascular disease (CAD) is the leading cause of death worldwide in women. Eight million women in the United States have heart disease. Although the prevalence of CAD in women is less than in men, women still die more often than men from the disease, and it is unknown whether this is due to the failure to identify the disease or the lack of appropriate treatment.[1] What is known is that 38% of women and 25% of men die after their first heart attack. Prevention is important in stopping this trend; however, once CAD is diagnosed many treatment options are available. Women have been underrepresented in cardiovascular studies, thus causing mixed information on the outcomes of different treatment options in women. This article reviews the current trials on revascularization strategies in women with stable coronary artery disease.

Even though CAD is the leading cause of death in both men and women, age-standardized mortality related to CAD has decreased by more than 40%, which is driven by a decline in mortality from the acute manifestations of CAD.[2,3] This reduction has been attributed to the emphasis on prevention and reduction of major risk factors as well as the improvement in medical treatment and revascularization.[4] Mortality from stable CAD, however, has not changed significantly over the last decade,[3] primarily because of an increase in chronic ischemic heart disease deriving from the reduction in mortality from the acute event.

## PATHOPHYSIOLOGY OF CAD IN WOMEN

Atherosclerosis is a progressive disorder of the vessel wall that promotes plaque buildup throughout the arterial system and also causes inflammation in the vessel, which leads to endothelial dysfunction, a common cause of cardiovascular morbidity and mortality in women.

The prevalence of obstructive coronary artery disease (stenosis >50%) is much less in women than in men. In a report from the American College of Cardiology's National Cardiovascular Data Registry (NCDR), 45% of the 375,886 patients referred for coronary angiography because of

[a] Section of Cardiology, Section of Cardiothoracic Surgery, University of Arizona, 1501 North Campbell Avenue, Tucson, AZ 85724, USA
[b] Cardiovascular Medicine, Detroit Medical Center, DMC Cardiovascular Institute, Wayne State University School of Medicine, 3990 John R Suite# 8362, Detroit, MI 48201, USA
* Corresponding author.
E-mail address: cgrines@dmc.org

Intervent Cardiol Clin 1 (2012) 165–172
doi:10.1016/j.iccl.2012.02.005
2211-7458/12/$ – see front matter © 2012 Elsevier Inc. All rights reserved.

stable chest pain were women. Across all age groups (<50 to ≥80 years), obstructive coronary disease was seen less in women than in men. For stenosis of 50% or more, this disease occurred in 27% to 64% of women and 45% to 87% of men. The prevalence of obstructive disease is very low in premenopausal women (5% in women aged <35 years) but does increase dramatically (to 79%) in women aged 75 years or older.

More than 60% of women with ischemic heart disease initially present with acute myocardial infarction (MI) or sudden cardiac death. Women, especially young women, are more likely to die from their coronary artery disease. The morphology of their acute event is more commonly caused by plaque erosion as opposed to plaque rupture, which is more commonly seen in men. Plaque rupture is characterized by a necrotic core

and a fibrous cap that is disrupted and becomes infiltrated by macrophages and lymphocytes. Women, especially younger women, more commonly present with plaque erosion, which is characterized by the absence of a fibrous cap and the exposure of vessel intima (**Fig. 1**).[5] When women have obstructive coronary disease they usually have atypical symptoms, including the following:

- Fatigue
- Shortness of breath
- Back pain
- Atypical chest pain.

Abundant data exist on revascularization strategies (percutaneous coronary intervention [PCI] vs coronary artery bypass grafting [CABG]) in the general population. Outcomes based on gender are less well known.

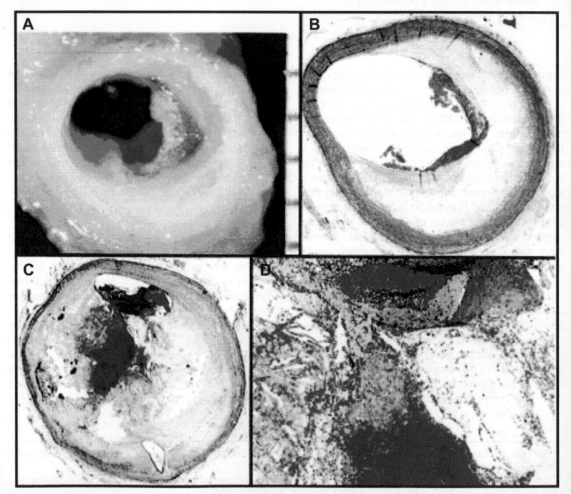

**Fig. 1.** (*A–D*) Plaque erosion with subocclusive thrombus. (*From* Bairey Merz CN, Shaw LJ, Bittner V, et al. Insights from the NHLBI-Sponsored Women's Ischemia Syndrome Evaluation (WISE) Study: Part II: gender differences in presentation, diagnosis, and outcome with regard to gender-based pathophysiology of atherosclerosis and macrovascular and microvascular coronary disease. J Am Coll Cardiol 2006;47(Suppl 3):S24; with permission.)

## REVASCULARIZATION STRATEGIES
### PCI: Women Versus Men

Women are underrepresented in research studies, and cardiology studies are no exception. Investigators now advocate for more studies that pay attention to gender differences and for a greater enrollment of women in existing studies. In the last decade, many of the large cardiology studies have reported gender outcomes. PCI has achieved standard-of-care status for acute coronary syndrome and ST-segment elevation MI. In the patient with stable coronary disease, the practice of routine PCI has been called into question with trials such as COURAGE (Clinical Outcomes Utilizing Revascularization and Aggressive Drug Evaluation) and SYNTAX (Synergy Between Percutaneous Coronary Intervention with TAXUS and Cardiac Surgery).[6,7] The ultimate goal of revascularization in stable coronary disease is to reduce the burden of ischemia, thus improving the quality of life by improving exercise capacity and reducing the amount of antianginals needed, while optically managing patients medically. This goal can be achieved by either PCI or CABG.

Although there have been no randomized controlled clinical studies looking particularly at gender differences in PCI outcomes on stable CAD, registry data and subgroup analysis are available from important large trials that do pay attention to this question. Shaw and colleagues[8] used the American College of Cardiology-NCDR, which is an angiographic database from more than 600 hospitals in the country, and found that there were higher in-hospital mortality rates for white women who presented with stable angina when compared with men (0.6% vs 0.5%, $P<.00001$), with no other differences noted for other ethnic populations. When considering the utilization rates for PCI and CABG, both were higher for men than for women across all ethnic subsets. The use of glycoprotein IIb/IIa inhibitors and aspirin were also lower in women than in men across all ethnic subsets ($P<.0001$). The decreased use of glycoprotein IIb/IIa inhibitors was mainly driven by less use of catheterization laboratory procedures for women than for men ($P<.0001$).

A few large trials have included gender differences in PCI outcomes as a substudy. Four of these trials may be considered outdated because they pertained to angioplasty only. In the current era most patients, if undergoing PCI, are stented. These angioplasty trials, however, are still worth mentioning. The earliest was the European CABRI (Coronary Angioplasty versus Bypass Revascularization Investigation) trial, which randomized 820 men and 234 women to CABG versus percutaneous transluminal coronary angioplasty (PTCA). Women, whether randomized to CABG or PTCA, had a higher risk of 1-year mortality than men (relative risk [RR] 2.07, 95% confidence interval [CI] 1.07–4.01, $P = .031$). Women also had more angina after 1 year in the PTCA group than men (RR 3.12, 95% CI 1.41–6.54, $P = .002$).[9]

The BARI (Bypass Angioplasty Revascularization Investigation) trial compared CABG with PTCA in patients with multivessel coronary disease. This study tested the hypothesis that patients with multivessel disease and severe angina or ischemia who underwent initial angioplasty did not do worse than those who underwent CABG. Of the 915 people who were enrolled, 249 were women. Women were more likely to undergo multilesion angioplasty (80% vs 76%, $P = .03$), and there was a trend toward women having more multivessel PTCA. Women also had a smaller reference vessel diameter than men.[10] At 5 years, there was no difference between men and women who were treated with PCI in survival and Q-wave MIs. However, women were more likely than men to have congestive heart failure (CHF) (4.8% vs 1.4%). Anginal status was similar between men and women for PTCA. The 10-year survival rates regarding PTCA between men and women were also similar. If undergoing PTCA, women were less likely than men to need repeat revascularization (RR 0.74, $P = .011$).[11]

Two other smaller studies, EAST (Emory Angioplasty versus Surgery Trial) and the GABI (German Angioplasty Bypass Surgery Investigation) trial, enrolled 103 women from 392 patients and 66 women from 359 patients, respectively. Both of these trials showed no difference in survival between men and women in either arm of the trials.[12,13]

In more current trials involving PCI with either bare metal stents (BMS) or drug-eluting stents (DES), results were similar. The SOS (Stent or Surgery) trial randomly compared CABG versus PCI with BMS in 206 women and 782 men with multivessel disease. Each patient was given a Seattle Angina Questionnaire (SAQ), and 6- and 12-month changes in physical limitation, angina frequency, and quality of life were assessed. At the time of revascularization, women were older, more ill, and had lower SAQ scores than men. After PCI with a BMS, both men and women had significant improvements in all 3 categories of the SAQ. However, CABG was clearly more beneficial than PCI in men in the 3 categories. The results were different in women. At 6 months, there was more benefit of CABG than PCI in the health status of women, but at 1 year, the status of the PCI group equaled that of the CABG group.[14]

In the MASS II (Medicine, Angioplasty, or Surgery Study) trial, 611 patients including 196 women were randomly assigned to CABG, PCI, or medical treatment. Considering gender as a subgroup analysis, investigators found that for the primary end point of death, MI, and angina requiring mechanical revascularization, PCI was more beneficial than optimal medical therapy (OMT) (hazard ratio [HR] 1.57, 95% CI 1.01–2.46, $P = .047$).[15] The COURAGE trial randomized 2287 patients including 338 women to OMT with PCI or OMT alone. Although there was no difference in any end point between OMT or OMT with PCI, the subgroup analysis showed there was a trend toward OMT with PCI for women (HR 0.65, 95% CI 0.4–1.06, $P = .03$) in the reduction of death or MI.[6] The SYNTAX trial did not analyze gender as a subgroup; however, when the investigators looked at 1-year major adverse cardiovascular and cerebrovascular event (MACCE) rates in patients with left main disease, they found that female gender was a significant predictor of events (odds ratio [OR] 0.50, 95% CI 0.27–0.91, $P = .02$).[7]

Most trials from this decade that have evaluated percutaneous revascularization outcomes comparing women with men have shown no difference in the in-hospital major adverse cardiac event (MACE), CABG, and death rates.[16–19] The largest representative study was from the Mayo clinic, which retrospectively looked at 18,885 consecutive patients in 2 time periods, 1979 to 1995 and 1996 to 2004. The primary end points were 30-day mortality and long-term mortality. In the first period there were 7904 patients and in the second, 10,981 patients. Twenty-eight percent were women in the first period and 31% were women in the second period. Once again, women were shown to be older and with more comorbid conditions such as hypertension, diabetes, or hypercholesterolemia. The 30-day mortality for women and men was 4.4% and 2.8%, respectively in the early group and 2.9% and 2.2%, respectively, in the later group. There was a significant decrease in the 30-day mortality between the early and later groups of women and men ($P = .002$, $P = .04$). Long-term survival, however, was similar between the early and later groups of both women and men. There was also no difference between women and men in the early or later group regarding in-hospital events or MI.[16]

## Stent Trials

A few trials, of which TAXUS-IV was the first, have specifically investigated DES placement and outcomes in women and men. Lansky and colleagues[20] sought to determine whether gender influenced the results of implanting paclitaxel-eluting stents. A total of 1314 patients were randomized to TAXUS (DES-paclitaxel) stents versus EXPRESS (Early Use of Existing Preventive Strategies for Stroke [bare metal]) stents. In the TAXUS cohort, 187 of the 662 patients were women and in the EXPRESS cohort, 180 of the 652 patients were women. The primary end point was the rate of ischemia-driven target vessel revascularization (TVR). Other end points were death, MI, target lesion revascularization (TLR), target vessel failure, stent thrombosis, and MACE. The results showed that women were older and had more comorbidities, such as diabetes, hypertension, renal insufficiency, and unstable angina, than men. Female gender was not a predictor of TLR or TVR (OR 1.72, 95% CI 0.68–4.62, $P = .25$). There were lower rates of MI, TLR, and MACE in women who were randomized to the TAXUS stent. There was no difference between men and women in the end points for TAXUS stent.

Solinas and colleagues[21] analyzed gender-specific outcomes after sirolimus-eluting stent (SES) implantation, which was a pooled analysis from 4 different randomized SES versus BMS trials. These trials were RAVEL (Randomized Comparison of a Sirolimus-Eluting Stent with a Standard Stent for Coronary Revascularization),[22] SIRIUS (SIRolImUS-coated Bx Velocity balloon expandable stent in the treatment of patients with de novo coronary artery lesions),[23] E-SIRIUS (Sirolimus-eluting stents for treatment of patients with long atherosclerotic lesions in small coronary arteries),[24] and C-SIRIUS (Canadian study of the sirolimus-eluting stent in the treatment of patients with long de novo lesions in small native coronary arteries).[25] In total 1748 patients were enrolled, 497 of whom women. The end points were identical for all 4 trials. MACE was defined as death, MI, and TVR. TLR was also an end point. In this analysis, similar to TAXUS-IV, investigators found that women were older and more frequently had type 2 diabetes mellitus, hypertension, and CHF. Overall clinical outcomes were similar between men and women. There was a significant 1-year reduction in MACE rates (66.7%) for both genders driven by a decrease in TLR and TVR. Treatment with SES was also associated with a decrease of in-segment binary restenosis in both women (6.3% vs 43.8%, $P<.0001$) and men (6.4% vs 35.6%, $P<.0001$). The favorable outcomes of SES implantation were independent of gender.[21]

Another study specifically involved stent implantation and gender in patients with their first manifestation of coronary disease, including stable disease and acute coronary syndromes. This study was a small one, looking at all mTOR-inhibitor

DES (sirolimus-, zotarolimus-, and everolimus-eluting stents), which enrolled 138 consecutive patients including 40 women. The end point was MACE, defined as cardiac death, MI, and clinically driven TLR at 12 months. MACE occurred more frequently in women than in men (25% vs 11%, $P = .05$). The study concludes that women may have a worse outcome than men with the implantation of mTOR-inhibitor DES.[26] This study was not supported by other larger trials.

The last, and most recent, study was a subset analysis from the SPIRIT III randomized clinical trial. This study looked at 1001 patients with coronary artery lesions up to 28 mm in length in 2.5- to 3.75-mm diameter vessels. These patients were prospectively randomized to receive XIENCE V (everolimus-eluting) stents or TAXUS (paclitaxel-eluting) stents. Six hundred and sixty-nine patients (30% women) were randomized to XIENCE V and 332 (34% women) were randomized to TAXUS. In this subgroup analysis, women had higher 3-year MACE rates and higher TLR rates than men (16.0% vs 10.0%, $P = .01$ and 10.2% vs 5.3%, $P = .008$). Women who had XIENCE V did have much lower MACE rates and lower TLR rates than those women who received TAXUS (12.2% vs 22.6%, $P = .03$ and 16.0% vs 26.4%, $P = .03$, respectively). Stent thrombosis and bleeding complication rates were similar between the 2 groups and between women and men. The investigators hypothesized that the MACE and TLR rates might have been higher in women because there was prespecified follow-up in all patients. Women tend to have vague symptoms and might not always be evaluated. In this study they were all reevaluated.[27]

## CABG

Unlike the situation with PCI, being a woman is an independent risk factor for morbidity and mortality in patients undergoing CABG. Women have a higher risk of morbidity, higher mortality, and experience less relief from angina than men, even though they make up less than 30% of the CABG population.[28,29] The reasons for this are still being elucidated. Women have smaller coronary arteries, but this alone cannot account for the increase in morbidity and mortality, and women have fewer bypass grafts and have underutilization of the internal mammary artery. The fact that women are usually older and need urgent revascularization with CABG may play a role in the increase in worse outcomes for women. Older age is associated with an increase in comorbid conditions such as diabetes, hypertension, hypercholesterolemia, CHF, and cerebrovascular disease

(**Box 1**).[30,31] Body-surface area (BSA) has also been seen as a risk factor for morbidity and mortality. BSA of less than 1.6 $m^2$ is associated with increased mortality despite gender. Women are known to have smaller BSA, and this correlates well with smaller coronary artery diameter and reduced graft patency.[32] If one controls for older age, diabetes, and valvular disease, female gender is still an independent risk factor for mortality in cardiac surgery (3.81% vs 2.43% for men).[31]

Women have worse 30-day outcomes after CABG (**Table 1**).[33] Poor outcomes range from problems with postoperative MI to longer ventilation requirements, sepsis, sternal wound infections, and need for pressors. These outcomes could be related to older age and the increased number of comorbid conditions women have when undergoing CABG. Alam and colleagues[34] also reported poor postoperative outcomes in a recent study of 13,115 patients of whom 3267 were women. Even after propensity matching, there was still an increased risk of postoperative mortality for women (OR 1.84, 95% CI 1.22–2.78).

---

**Box 1**
**Common risk factors per gender**

*Preoperative risk factors in women*

Older age at presentation

Angina class III or IV

Urgent surgical interventions

Preoperative intra-aortic balloon pump usage

Congestive heart failure

Previous percutaneous transluminal coronary angioplasty

Diabetes mellitus

Hypertension

Peripheral vascular disease

Smaller body surface area

Lower hematocrit

*Preoperative risk factors in men*

Ejection fraction less than 35%

Three-vessel disease

Repeat operations

Recent significant history of smoking

Renal failure

Chronic obstructive pulmonary disease

*From* Blasberg JD, Schwartz GS, Balaram SK. The role of gender in coronary surgery. Eur J Cardiothorac Surg 2011;40(3):715–21; with permission.

## Table 1
## Summary of 30-day mortality studies

| Authors | N | Year | Mortality (Men vs Women) |
|---|---|---|---|
| Abramov et al[28] | 4823 | 2002 | 2.7% vs 1.8% ($P = .09$) |
| Aldea et al[35] | 1743 | 1999 | 1.5% vs 1.0% ($P = .33$) |
| Blankstein et al[31] | 15440 | 2005 | 4.24% vs 2.23% ($P<.0001$) |
| Carey et al[36] | 1335 | 1995 | 6.3% vs 3.1% ($P = .011$) |
| Christakis et al[37] | 7025 | 1995 | 3.5% vs 1.8% ($P<.0001$) |
| Doenst et al[38] | 1567 | 2006 | 7% vs 4% ($P = .026$) |
| Edwards et al[29] | 344913 | 1998 | 4.52% vs 2.61% ($P<.001$) |
| Hammar et al[39] | 3933 | 1997 | 3.0% vs 1.7% ($P<.01$) |
| Humphries et al[40] | 25212 | 2007 | 3.6% vs 2.0% ($P<.001$) |
| Koch et al[41] | 15597 | 2003 | 2.4% vs 1.4% ($P<.01$) |
| O'Connor et al[42] | 3055 | 1993 | 7.1% vs 3.3% ($P<.001$) |
| Ramstrom et al[43] | 220 | 1993 | 5.6% vs 2.4% ($P<.001$) |
| Vaccarino et al[44] | 15178 | 2002 | 5.3% vs 2.9% ($P<.001$) |
| Woods et al[45] | 5324 | 2003 | 3.16% vs 1.95% ($P = .007$) |

*From* Blasberg JD, Schwartz GS, Balaram SK. The role of gender in coronary surgery. Eur J Cardiothorac Surg 2011; 40(3):715–21; with permission.

When discussing revascularization strategies, even though with CABG women have higher morbidity and mortality than men, it is still an option. For women with stable CAD who need revascularization, CABG was no better than PCI, but better than OMT in the MASS II trial regarding the primary end point (death, MI, angina requiring mechanical revascularization) at 10 years (HR 0.43, 95% CI 0.31–0.60, $P = .001$).[15] This was also seen in the SOS trial in which improvements in the SAQ score were statistically significant for CABG over PCI at 6 months, but by 1 year there was no difference in SAQ scores for women.[14]

## SUMMARY

Over the last decade there has been more focus on understanding gender differences regarding CAD and its treatment. Even though women are less likely than men to have obstructive CAD, women have more angina and die of CAD more often. In women with stable CAD, PCI has emerged as an appropriate revascularization strategy that does not seem to put them at increased risk. Despite being older, having more comorbidities including diabetes, and smaller vessels that are at risk for restenosis, outcomes between men and women treated with stents appear to be similar. Such is not the case with CABG; however, women have fewer left internal mammary artery grafts, more immediate postoperative complications, and higher mortality than men. More studies enrolling larger numbers of women are needed to better define the best treatment options for women with coronary disease.

## REFERENCES

1. Mosca L, Banka CL, Benjamin EJ, et al. Evidence-based guidelines for cardiovascular disease prevention in women: 2007 update. Circulation 2007; 115(11):1481–501.
2. Lloyd-Jones D, Adams R, Carnethon M, et al. Heart disease and stroke statistics—2009 update: a report from the American Heart Association Statistics Committee and Stroke Statistics Subcommittee. Circulation 2009;119(3):480–6.
3. Boersma E, Mercado N, Poldermans D, et al. Acute myocardial infarction. Lancet 2003;361(9360):847–58.
4. Ford ES, Ajani UA, Croft JB, et al. Explaining the decrease in U.S. deaths from coronary disease, 1980-2000. N Engl J Med 2007;356(23):2388–98.
5. Bairey Merz CN, Shaw LJ, Bittner V, et al. Insights from the NHLBI-Sponsored Women's Ischemia Syndrome Evaluation (WISE) Study: Part II: gender differences in presentation, diagnosis, and outcome with regard to gender-based pathophysiology of atherosclerosis and macrovascular and microvascular coronary disease. J Am Coll Cardiol 2006; 47(Suppl 3):S21–9.
6. Boden WE, O'Rourke RA, Teo KK, et al. Optimal medical therapy with or without PCI for stable coronary disease. N Engl J Med 2007;356(15):1503–16.
7. Morice MC, Serruys PW, Kappetein AP, et al. Outcomes in patients with de novo left main disease treated with either percutaneous coronary intervention using paclitaxel-eluting stents or coronary artery bypass graft treatment in the Synergy Between Percutaneous Coronary Intervention with TAXUS and Cardiac Surgery (SYNTAX) trial. Circulation 2010;121(24):2645–53.
8. Shaw LJ, Shaw RE, Merz CN, et al. Impact of ethnicity and gender differences on angiographic coronary artery disease prevalence and in-hospital mortality in the American College of Cardiology-National Cardiovascular Data Registry. Circulation 2008;117(14):1787–801.

9. First-year results of CABRI (Coronary Angioplasty versus Bypass Revascularisation Investigation). CABRI Trial Participants. Lancet 1995;346(8984): 1179–84.

10. Jacobs AK, Kelsey SF, Brooks MM, et al. Better outcome for women compared with men undergoing coronary revascularization: a report from the bypass angioplasty revascularization investigation (BARI). Circulation 1998;98(13):1279–85.

11. BARI Investigators. The final 10-year follow-up results from the BARI randomized trial. J Am Coll Cardiol 2007;49(15):1600–6.

12. King SB 3rd, Kosinski AS, Guyton RA, et al. Eight-year mortality in the Emory Angioplasty versus Surgery Trial (EAST). J Am Coll Cardiol 2000;35(5): 1116–21.

13. Kaehler J, Koester R, Billman W, et al. 13-year follow-up of the German angioplasty bypass surgery investigation. Eur Heart J 2005;26(20):2148–53.

14. Zhang Z, Weintraub WS, Mahoney EM, et al. Relative benefit of coronary artery bypass grafting versus stent-assisted percutaneous coronary intervention for angina pectoris and multivessel coronary disease in women versus men (one-year results from the Stent or Surgery trial). Am J Cardiol 2004;93(4): 404–9.

15. Hueb W, Lopes N, Gersh BJ, et al. Ten-year follow-up survival of the Medicine, Angioplasty, or Surgery Study (MASS II): a randomized controlled clinical trial of 3 therapeutic strategies for multivessel coronary artery disease. Circulation 2010;122(10): 949–57.

16. Singh M, Rihal CS, Gersh BJ, et al. Mortality differences between men and women after percutaneous coronary interventions. A 25-year, single-center experience. J Am Coll Cardiol 2008;51(24):2313–20.

17. Thompson CA, Kaplan AV, Friedman BJ, et al. Gender-based differences of percutaneous coronary intervention in the drug-eluting stent era. Catheter Cardiovasc Interv 2006;67(1):25–31.

18. Abbott JD, Vlachos HA, Selzer F, et al. Gender-based outcomes in percutaneous coronary intervention with drug-eluting stents (from the National Heart, Lung, and Blood Institute Dynamic Registry). Am J Cardiol 2007;99(5):626–31.

19. Nowakowska-Arendt A, Grabczewska Z, Kozinski M, et al. Gender differences and in-hospital mortality in patients undergoing percutaneous coronary interventions. Kardiol Pol 2008;66(6):632–9 [discussion: 640–1].

20. Lansky AJ, Costa RA, Mooney M, et al. Gender-based outcomes after paclitaxel-eluting stent implantation in patients with coronary artery disease. J Am Coll Cardiol 2005;45(8):1180–5.

21. Solinas E, Nikolsky E, Lansky AJ, et al. Gender-specific outcomes after sirolimus-eluting stent implantation. J Am Coll Cardiol 2007;50(22):2111–6.

22. Morice MC, Serruys PW, Sousa JE, et al. A randomized comparison of a sirolimus-eluting stent with a standard stent for coronary revascularization. N Engl J Med 2002;346(23):1773–80.

23. Moses JW, Leon MB, Popma JJ, et al. Sirolimus-eluting stents versus standard stents in patients with stenosis in a native coronary artery. N Engl J Med 2003;349(14):1315–23.

24. Schofer J, Schlüter M, Gershlick AH, et al. Sirolimus-eluting stents for treatment of patients with long atherosclerotic lesions in small coronary arteries: double-blind, randomised controlled trial (E-SIRIUS). Lancet 2003;362(9390):1093–9.

25. Schampaert E, Cohen EA, Schlüter M, et al. The Canadian study of the sirolimus-eluting stent in the treatment of patients with long de novo lesions in small native coronary arteries (C-SIRIUS). J Am Coll Cardiol 2004;43(6):1110–5.

26. Niccoli G, Sgueglia GA, Cosentino N, et al. Impact of gender on clinical outcomes after mTOR-inhibitor drug-eluting stent implantation in patients with first manifestation of ischaemic heart disease. Eur J Cardiovasc Prev Rehabil 2011. [Epub ahead of print].

27. Ng VG, Lansky AJ, Hermiller JB, et al. Three-year results of safety and efficacy of the everolimus-eluting coronary stent in women (from the SPIRIT III randomized clinical trial). Am J Cardiol 2011;107(6):841–8.

28. Abramov D, Tamariz MG, Sever JY, et al. The influence of gender on the outcome of coronary artery bypass surgery. Ann Thorac Surg 2000;70(3): 800–5 [discussion: 806].

29. Edwards FH, Carey JS, Grover FL, et al. Impact of gender on coronary bypass operative mortality. Ann Thorac Surg 1998;66(1):125–31.

30. Sharoni E, Kogan A, Medalion B, et al. Is gender an independent risk factor for coronary bypass grafting? Thorac Cardiovasc Surg 2009;57(4):204–8.

31. Blankstein R, Ward RP, Arnsdorf M, et al. Female gender is an independent predictor of operative mortality after coronary artery bypass graft surgery: contemporary analysis of 31 Midwestern hospitals. Circulation 2005;112(Suppl 9):I323–7.

32. O'Connor NJ, Morton JR, Birkmeyer JD, et al. Effect of coronary artery diameter in patients undergoing coronary bypass surgery. Northern New England Cardiovascular Disease Study Group. Circulation 1996;93(4):652–5.

33. Blasberg JD, Schwartz GS, Balaram SK. The role of gender in coronary surgery. Eur J Cardiothorac Surg 2011;40(3):715–21.

34. Alam M, Elayda MA, Shahzad SA, et al. Association of gender with morbidity and mortality after isolated coronary artery bypass grafting. A propensity score matched analysis. Int J Cardiol 2012. [Epub ahead of print].

35. Aldea GS, Gaudiani JM, Shapira OM, et al. Effect of gender on postoperative outcomes and hospital

stays after coronary artery bypass grafting. Ann Thorac Surg 1999;67:1097–103.

36. Carey JS, Cukingnan RA, Singer L. Health status after myocardial revascularization: inferior results in women. Ann Thor Surg 1995;59(1):112–7.

37. Christakis GT, Weisel RD, Buth KJ, et al. Is body size the cause for poor outcomes of coronary artery bypass operations in women? J Thorac Cardiovasc Surg 1995;110:1344–56.

38. Doenst T, Ivanov J, Borger MA, et al. Sex-specific long-term outcomes after combined valve and coronary artery surgery. Ann Thorac Surg 2006;81: 1632–6.

39. Hammar N, Sandberg E, Larsen FF, et al. Comparison of early and late mortality in men and women after isolated coronary artery bypass graft surgery in Stockholm, Sweden, 1980 to 1989. J Am Coll Cardiol 1997;29(3):659–64.

40. Humphries KH, Gao M, Pu A, et al. Significant improvement in short-term mortality in women undergoing coronary artery bypass surgery (1991–2004). J Am Coll Cardiol 2007;49:1552–8.

41. Koch CG, Khandwala F, Nussmeier N, et al. Gender and outcomes after coronary artery bypass grafting: a propensity-matched comparison. J Thorac Cardiovasc Surg 2003;126:2032–43.

42. O'Connor GT, Morton JR, Diehl MJ, et al. Differences between men and women in hospital mortality associated with coronary artery bypass graft surgery. Circulation 1993;88(Pt 1):2104–10.

43. Ramstrom J, Lund O, Cadavid E, et al. Multiarterial coronary artery bypass grafting with special reference to small vessel disease and results in women. Eur Heart J 1993;14:634–9.

44. Vaccarino V, Abramson JL, Veledar E, et al. Sex differences in hospital mortality after coronary artery bypass surgery: evidence for a higher mortality in younger women. Circulation 2002;105: 1176–81.

45. Woods SE, Noble G, Smith JM, et al. The influence of gender in patients undergoing coronary artery bypass graft surgery: an eight-year prospective hospitalized cohort study. J Am Coll Surg 2003; 196:428–34.

# Interventional Management of ACS in Women: STEMI and NSTEMI

Nitish Naik, MD[a], Ambuj Roy, MD[a],
Annapoorna S. Kini, MD, MRCP[b],*

## KEYWORDS

- ST elevation myocardial infarction
- Acute coronary syndromes • Percutaneous intervention
- Non–ST elevation myocardial infarction

Coronary heart disease (CHD) is the leading cause of morbidity and mortality in women. The prevalence of CHD in women older than 20 years was 6.1% as per 2008 US data.[1] Although there has been a steady decline in cardiovascular deaths, in the year 2007 there were approximately 190,300 deaths secondary to CHD in women.[2] Cardiovascular deaths, however, still account for more deaths than many other leading causes, such as cancer, chronic lower respiratory disease, Alzheimer disease, and accidents combined. From the year 1984, more women than men have died because of cardiovascular diseases. Despite these disconcerting data, women and physicians continue to underestimate the significant community burden of CHD. In a study published in 2002, only 8% to 22% of women were aware that among them coronary artery disease (CAD) was the leading cause of death.[3] Similarly, in a national survey on physician awareness conducted across various states in the United States, less than 20% of physicians were cognizant of the contribution of cardiovascular deaths to overall mortality in women.[4]

Percutaneous interventions (PCI) have increasingly played a crucial role in management of most patients presenting with ST elevation myocardial infarction (STEMI) and also for patients with unstable angina (UA) or non-STEMI (NSTEMI). Efficacy of these interventions over pharmacologic therapy in restoring patency of diseased coronary arteries, preventing reocclusion, and preserving myocardial function has been well proved in numerous trials. Current guidelines strongly support an interventional approach for patients presenting with STEMI.[5,6] For patients presenting with UA/NSTEMI an interventional approach is still recommended with some caveats.[7,8] However, despite proved benefits, use of PCIs is still markedly lower in women; of the 1.3 million procedures performed in the United States in 2007, only 33% were performed in women.[1] This article reviews the role of PCIs in management of STEMI and UA/NSTEMI in women.

## THE GENDER GAP

The clinical presentation and pattern of CAD varies between the genders. Women are likely to be older and have more comorbidities, such as diabetes, hypertension, and heart failure.[9] They are more likely than men to present with atypical symptoms and UA.[10] They are likely to face greater delays in diagnosis of CHD than men and are less likely to receive appropriate investigations and therapy at admission and discharge.[11,12] Women are more likely to have normal angiograms despite more anginal symptoms. Prevalence of multivessel disease including left main disease is also lower in women, despite higher prevalence of risk factors. Their coronary arteries are smaller than in men (mean diameter of 2.9 mm vs 3.09 mm, respectively).[13] Despite a lesser

a Department of Cardiology, All India Institute of Medical Sciences, Ansari Nagar, New Delhi 110029, India
b Mount Sinai School of Medicine, One Gustave L. Levy Place, Box 1030, New York, NY 10029–6574, USA
* Corresponding author.
E-mail address: annapoorna.kini@mountsinai.org

Intervent Cardiol Clin 1 (2012) 173–182
doi:10.1016/j.iccl.2012.02.002

burden of atherosclerotic CAD, more women die of their first MI than men.[14] Their unadjusted mortality and bleeding and vascular complication rates after PCIs are also higher than in men.[11] However, although this was previously an area of controversy,[15] a large risk-adjusted analysis by Kovacic and coworkers[9] clarified that gender is not an independent predictor of mortality after PCI in the drug eluting stent (DES) era. In turn, this has now placed added emphasis on attention to risk factors in females undergoing PCI.[16]

## STEMI

Acute coronary syndromes (ACS) and STEMI accounted for 370,000 events annually among women in the United States in the year 2007.[1] There has been a steady decline in the incidence of STEMI in United States; the National Registry of Myocardial Infarction 4 reported that STEMIs account for only 29% of all MIs.[17] In a more recent study that analyzed population trends in MI from 1999 to 2008, the incidence of MI declined steadily from 133 cases per 100,000 person-years in 1999 to 50 cases per 100,000 patient-years in 2008.[18]

### Fibrinolysis

There are no gender-specific differences in the evaluation and treatment of female patients with STEMI, even though women have been underrepresented in all published trials. Although primary PCI is the preferred revascularization strategy for patients with STEMI, a sizable proportion of patients still receive fibrinolytic therapy. Although women receiving fibrinolysis have higher unadjusted mortality than men because of more risk factors, such as diabetes, heart failure, hypertension, and older age, they still continue to face not only longer delays in diagnosis of STEMI but unfortunately also greater in-hospital delays than men in the administration of fibrinlolysis.[19–21] These disparities in clinical care have persisted despite programs designed to enhance delivery of evidence-based care among hospitalized patients. However, after adjusting for these variables, no gender difference in mortality is appreciable in some studies.[22] In the GUSTO IIb trial, which included 3662 women, there was a nonsignificant trend toward higher mortality and reinfarction after adjusting for these baseline factors.[20] However, some studies have reported a higher mortality in women despite correcting for baseline factors.[23]

### PCI

Results of primary angioplasty have been superior to fibrinolysis in the management of STEMI. In a trial on 395 patients comparing angioplasty with fibrinolysis, primary angioplasty was an independent predictor of survival in women.[21] The Gusto IIb trial revealed greater absolute benefit of primary PCI in women.[24] Primary angioplasty in women, compared with tissue plasminogen activator, prevented 56 additional events per 1000 women treated as against 42 additional events prevented per 1000 men treated. Thus, despite similar odds reduction of primary angioplasty over fibrinolysis for men and women, the number needed to treat to prevent an adverse event was smaller for women compared with men because of a higher event rate in women. Primary angioplasty followed by coronary stenting affords similar benefits in genders.[25] In the multicentric CADILLAC trial, primary stenting significantly reduced the 1-year major adverse cardiac events and target vessel revascularization.

### Current Recommendations

The American College of Cardiology/American Heart Association and the European Society of Cardiology do not advocate any separate gender-specific recommendations for evaluating and treating women with STEMI.[5,6]

## NSTEMI

UA and NSTEMI together constitute most ACS events in developed countries. In the Worcester study, the proportion of NSTEMI increased progressively from 0.02% to 0.13% from 1975 to 1997.[26] The reason behind this epidemiologic variation in clinical presentation of ACS is probably multifactorial; better risk factor control, increasing use of aspirin and statins, and earlier recognition and treatment of CAD have all contributed in varying measures.

### Early Invasive Versus Conservative Management Strategies

Numerous trials have evaluated the role of PCIs in management of male and female patients with UA/NSTEMI. Early trials, such as the Thrombolysis in Myocardial Ischemia (TIMI) IIIB trial, evaluated the role of thrombolytic therapy in patients with NSTEMI, which was soon abandoned because of poor efficacy and more adverse events in patients receiving thrombolytic therapy.[27] This was followed by trials that examined a strategy of routine early intervention in all patients with UA/NSTEMI versus a strategy of conservative management and selective invasive therapy in patients who either failed medical therapy or had positive stress tests requiring revascularization. These trials excluded patients who were at very high risk for ischemic events, such as patients with refractory ischemia, hemodynamic instability, and ventricular arrhythmias, who underwent early angiography and revascularization as appropriate. The VANQWISH (Veterans Affairs Non-Q Wave Infarction Strategies in Hospital),[28] FRISC 2 (Fragmin and Fast Revascularization during Instability in CAD),[29] and RITA 3 (Randomized Intervention Trial of UA)[30] are three early trials that investigated such a strategy. They were followed by the TACTICS–TIMI 18 (Treat Angina with Aggrastat and Determine Cost of Therapy with an Invasive or Conservative Strategy),[31] VINO (Value of First Day Angiography/Angioplasty in Evolving Non-ST Segment Elevation Myocardial Infarction),[32] ICTUS (Invasive vs Conservative Treatment in Unstable Coronary Syndromes),[33] and OASIS 5 (Organization to Assess Strategies in Acute Ischemic Syndromes)[34] studies. Gender-specific outcomes were separately analyzed in some of these trials (FRISC II, RITA 3, TACTCIS-TIMI 18, ICTUS, and OASIS 5 trials).

## Gender-Based Differences

Two of these earlier trials, the FRISC II[35] and RITA 3,[36] reported a higher cardiovascular event rate in women randomized to a routine early invasive therapy even though the overall results supported an early invasive approach over a conservative strategy. In the FRISC II trial, 2457 patients (749 women and 1708 men) were randomized to an early invasive or conservative strategy. All patients received aspirin and were randomized to either dalteparin or placebo. Patients in the early invasive arm underwent coronary angiograms within a few days, whereas revascularization procedures were scheduled within a week from randomization. Overall, revascularization was performed in 77% (PCI in 42% and coronary artery bypass graft [CABG] in 35%) of patients in the early invasive arm and 37% (PCI in 17% and CABG in 18%) of patients in the conservative arm. The trial reported a significant reduction in the composite primary end point of death or MI in the early invasive group compared with the selective invasive group (9.4% vs 12.1%, respectively). However, on subgroup analysis, the trial did not find any difference in death or MI at 1 year between the two groups in women. This was in contrast to the results in men, in whom an invasive strategy was associated with a significant reduction in the primary end point in the invasive group compared with the conservative group (9.6% vs 15.8%, respectively) **(Fig. 1)**.

The RITA 3 trial reported unfavorable results with a routine early invasive strategy in women. This trial

was conducted between November 1997 and October 2001 across 45 centers in England and Scotland and enrolled 1810 patients (692 women) with UA/NSTEMI who were randomized to early invasive or conservative therapy. In general, women compared with men were a little older, had more anginal symptoms, were more likely to be hypertensive, and had higher levels of cholesterol. All patients received aspirin and enoxaparin. Among patients randomized to the early invasive arm, 97% underwent a coronary angiogram within a median of 2 days. Burden of CAD was lower in women, as reflected by absence of significant disease in 37% of women (compared with 12% of men). Revascularization was performed in 58% of patients in the intervention arm (PCI in 36%, CABG in 22%). Although PCI was performed in a similar proportion of men and women, CABG was performed in only 12% of women (compared with 30% of men). There was a significant reduction in the primary end point of death or MI or refractory angina in the early invasive group compared with the conservative group (9.6% vs 14.5%, respectively). However, the trial reported a differential effect of gender on the outcome of death or MI with the two strategies. Although men fared better with an early invasive approach, no benefit was observed among women **(Fig. 2)**. When stratified into low-, moderate-, and high-risk groups depending on the TIMI risk score, higher event rates were still observed in women in the moderate- and high-risk groups.

In contrast to the previously mentioned trials, the TACTIS-TIMI 18 trial supported a routine early invasive approach in men and women.[37] This was a randomized trial that evaluated an early invasive versus conservative strategy in 2220 patients who presented with UA or NSTEMI. One third of the patients recruited in the trials were women. In contrast to the previous two trials, all patients in this trial had elevated levels of cardiac troponin. In addition to aspirin and intravenous unfractionated heparin, all patients received the GPIIbIIIa inhibitor, tirofiban. Patients in the early invasive arm underwent revascularization at a mean of 22 hours after randomization. Nearly 44% of the patients randomized to the conservative arm also received a revascularization procedure within 6 months of randomization. A significant reduction in the primary end point of death, MI, or rehospitalization for an acute coronary syndrome was observed in the early invasive arm compared with the conservative arm (15.9% vs 19.4%, respectively). This trial demonstrated a 28% odds reduction in the primary end point of death, MI, or rehospitalization for ACS among women randomized to an early invasive strategy (17% incidence

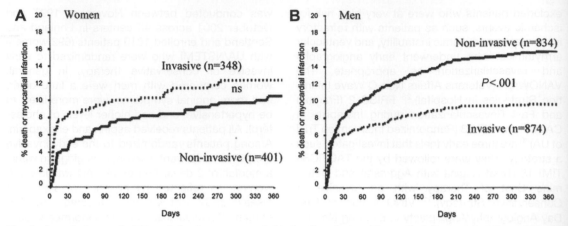

**Fig. 1.** Cumulative probability of death or myocardial infarction during 12-month follow-up in (*A*) women and (*B*) men in relation to randomized strategy (*solid line*, noninvasive strategy; *dotted line*, early invasive strategy). ns, not significant. (*From* Lagerqvist B, Säfström K, Ståhle E, et al. FRISC II Study Group Investigators. Is early invasive treatment of unstable coronary artery disease equally effective for both women and men? FRISC II Study Group Investigators. J Am Coll Cardiol 2001;38:41–8; with permission.)

of the primary end point among patients in early invasive arm vs 19.6% in patients in conservative arm). This benefit was further enhanced in the subgroup of women with elevated troponin T (19% in early invasive group vs 29% in conservative arm) (**Fig. 3**).

Another study that also supported the role of routine early invasive strategy in both genders presenting with UA/NSTEMI was an observational study conducted on 1450 consecutive patients (417 women) presenting with ACS.[13] Coronary angiography with subsequent revascularization was performed within 24 hours as per a prespecified protocol. Most patients underwent percutaneous revascularization (PCI/CABG ratio of 5:1 in women and 4:1 in men). This was in sharp contrast to the ratio

in the FRISC trial where the ratio was nearly 1:1. The primary end point of death or MI occurred in 7% of women compared with 10.5% in men (*P* = .045) with women having a more favorable outcome than men at a mean follow-up of 20 months.

The ICTUS trial also did not report any gender-based difference in outcomes between the two strategies on subgroup analysis.[33] This trial enrolled 1200 patients (320 women) with UA/NSTEMI who had elevated cardiac troponin and randomized them to an early invasive strategy or selective invasive strategy. All patients were treated with aspirin and received enoxaparin for 48 hours. Patients scheduled for PCI also received abciximab. Revascularization was performed in 76% of the early invasive group and 40% in the

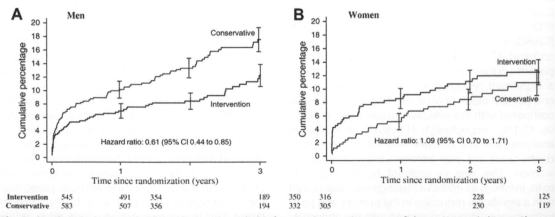

**Fig. 2.** (*A, B*) Cumulative risk of death or myocardial infarction by gender. CI, confidence interval. (*From* Clayton TC, Pocock SJ, Henderson RA, et al. Do men benefit more than women from an interventional strategy in patients with unstable angina or non-ST-elevation myocardial infarction? The impact of gender in the RITA 3 trial. Eur Heart J 2004;25:1641–50; with permission.)

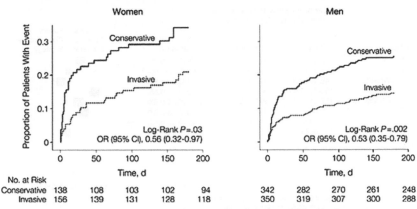

**Fig. 3.** Death, myocardial infarction, and rehospitalization for acute coronary syndrome in women and men with elevated troponin T levels, by strategy. Median follow-up time, 180 days for women and men. CI, confidence interval; OR, odds ratio. (*From* Glasser R, Herrmann HC, Murphy SA, et al. Benefit of an early invasive management strategy in women with acute coronary syndromes. JAMA 2002;288:3124–9; with permission.)

conservatively managed group during the initial hospitalization; the corresponding figures at 1 year were 79% and 54%, respectively. There was no difference in the composite primary end point of death, MI, or rehospitalization for angina at 1 year between the two strategies. On analyzing various subgroups, the authors did not report any difference in the primary outcome between the genders.

The OASIS 5 study, however, cautioned against the implementation of an early invasive approach in all patients.[34] Although there was no significant difference with regard to the rate of death, MI, or stroke in patients treated with either strategy, there was a trend toward higher mortality in women treated with an early invasive approach.

### Early Invasive Versus Late Invasive Management Strategies

Among patients in whom an early invasive strategy is selected for revascularization, clinical outcomes have been similar in men and women. The Timing of Intervention in Acute Coronary Syndromes (TIMACS) trial evaluated an early intervention strategy (median time to angiography after randomization of 14 hours) versus a delayed intervention strategy (median time of 50 hours) on outcomes in patients with UA/NSTEMI.[38] Although there was no difference in the primary outcome of death, MI, or stroke between the two strategies at 1 and 6 months, there was a significant reduction in the secondary end point of death, MI, or refractory ischemia in the early intervention group (9.5% vs 12.9% in the early and delayed intervention groups, respectively). On subgroup analysis, men and women had similar benefits on the secondary outcomes.

The contrasting results observed in women as against men in the FRISC II and RITA 3 trials could be caused by heterogeneity of the study population. Although gender-based outcomes was a predefined subgroup in these trials, the numbers of events were insufficient to draw firm conclusions. In the FRISC II trial, one of the factors that may have acted unfavorably against the invasive strategy in women versus men could have been the high mortality among women who underwent CABG (9.9% in women compared with 1.2% in men). In addition, the lower prevalence of angiographically significant CAD in women (nearly one-fourth of the women had normal coronaries, whereas another 31.9% had one-vessel disease) in FRISC II suggests inclusion of a low-risk study population that had less to gain from an invasive strategy. Similarly, the lack of benefit of a routine invasive strategy among women in the RITA 3 trial could be caused by several possibilities: less severe atherosclerotic obstructive disease, higher procedure-related complications in women, lower event rates in the conservative arm, referral bias, or a chance finding.

### Meta-Analyses

Because none of these trials were individually powered to analyze the effect of female gender on clinical outcomes, many meta-analyses have been performed to evaluate the preferred management strategy for women with UA/NSTEMI, incorporating the results of these trials. O'Donoghue and colleagues[39] conducted a meta-analysis that incorporated eight of the published randomized trials (3075 women and 7075 men). Although women had more baseline comorbidities, they still had less severe atherosclerotic CAD. A significant

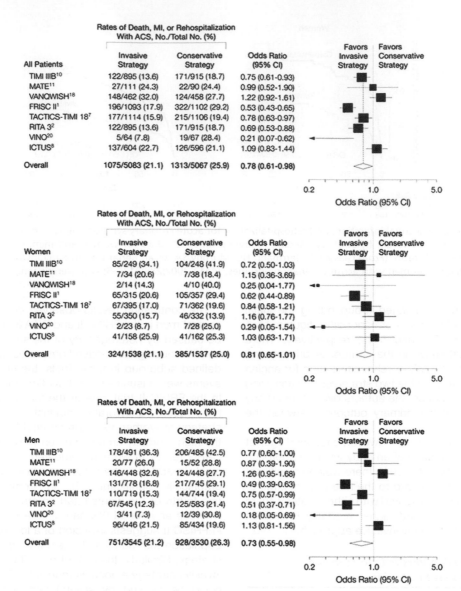

**Fig. 4.** Death, MI, or rehospitalization with ACS for biomarker status and ST-segment deviation in trials of an invasive versus conservative treatment strategy in NSTE ACS. CI, confidence interval; NSTE, non–ST-segment elevation. Odds ratios were generated from random-effects models. Size of data markers is weighted based on the inverse variance. The odds ratio (OR) and corresponding *P* value for the interaction terms for the efficacy of an invasive over a conservative strategy in biomarker-positive versus biomarker-negative patients were as follows: for all patients, OR, 0.79, *P* = .18; for women, OR, 0.75, *P* = .36; and for men, OR, 0.77, *P* = .09. The analogous data for patients with versus without ST-segment deviation were as follows: for all patients, OR, 0.83, *P* = .07; for women, OR, 0.87, *P* = .76; and for men, OR, 0.79, *P* = .07. VINO, VANQWISH, and ICTUS trials were excluded from the primary biomarker analysis because they only enrolled patients with elevated biomarkers, thus precluding the comparison of biomarker-positive and biomarker-negative subgroups. The meta-analysis OR and 95% CIs for the efficacy of an invasive strategy versus conservative strategy if those three trials were also included were as follows: for all patients biomarker-positive, OR, 0.72, 95% CI, 0.53–0.98; for all patients biomarker-negative, OR, 0.79, 95% CI, 0.60–1.03; for biomarker-positive men, OR, 0.71, 95% CI, 0.49–1.01; for biomarker-negative men, OR, 0.72, 95% CI, 0.54–0.98; for biomarker-positive women, OR, 0.71, 95% CI, 0.56–0.91; and for biomarker-negative women, OR, 0.94, 95% CI, 0.61–1.44. (*From* O'Donoghue M, Boden WE, Braunwald E, et al. Early invasive vs conservative treatment strategies in women and men with unstable angina and non-ST-segment elevation myocardial infarction: a meta-analysis. JAMA 2008;300:71–80; with permission.)

reduction in the composite end point of death, nonfatal MI, or rehospitalization with ACS was observed in the overall population in the invasive group compared with the conservatively managed patients (21.1% vs 25.9%, respectively; 95% confidence interval, 0.61–0.98) (**Fig. 4**). However, among women, benefit of an invasive strategy was observed only in troponin-positive women. In troponin-negative women, no significant benefit was observed with regard to the composite end point. The authors also reported a nonsignificant 35% higher odds ratio for the end point of death or MI among troponin-negative women randomized to the early invasive arm. The Cochrane database, in its meta-analyses, also indicated a significant reduction in the long-term risk of death or MI among women in the invasive arm (relative risk, 0.73; 95% confidence interval, 0.59–0.91).[40] In a meta-analysis of the FRISC II, RITA 3, and ICTUS trials that evaluated outcomes at 5 years, an early invasive strategy was associated with an 11.1% absolute risk reduction in occurrence of death or MI.[41] A smaller benefit was also seen in the low- and intermediate-risk groups (absolute risk reduction of 2%–3.8%). On univariate and multivariate analysis, gender was not predictive of worse outcomes.

However, another meta-analysis conducted by Swahn and colleagues,[34] which included the results of the OASIS 5 trial, reported no significant difference in the composite end point of death or MI between the two strategies. The authors, however, did not analyze the data further with regard to high-risk features, such as presence of positive biomarkers or ST segment deviation.

## Actual Practice Pattern

Actual practice patterns in the real world frequently differ from the results portrayed in randomized controlled trials. Morbidity and mortality figures are usually higher in the real world setting because sick patients are frequently excluded from randomized trials. The CRUSADE (Can Rapid Risk Stratification of Unstable Angina Patients Suppress Adverse Outcomes with Early Implementation of the ACC/AHA Guidelines) National Quality Improvement Initiative reported data on 40,912 patients (41% women) presenting with high-risk NSTEMI at nearly 400 US hospitals between March 2000 and December 2002.[42] Although women were older than men and more often had diabetes or hypertension, there were greater delays in diagnosis of an ACS in women than men. They were less likely to receive appropriate therapy at admission and discharge and were less likely to undergo cardiac catheterization. However, women were as likely as men to undergo revascularization once detected to have significant obstructive CAD. After adjustment for risk factors, women were not any more prone than men to adverse outcomes except for a higher risk of requiring transfusions. Even with implementation of various national programs to improve awareness about cardiovascular problems in women, the National Cardiovascular Data Registry Acute Coronary Treatment and Intervention Outcomes Network–Get with the Guidelines reported no further improvements in diagnostic and therapeutic delays in the community.[43]

## Current Recommendations

The European Society of Cardiology guidelines recommend similar evaluation and therapeutic strategies for both genders.[8] The American College of Cardiology Foundation/American Heart Association guidelines recommend risk stratification in deciding the appropriate therapeutic strategy: an early invasive strategy for women presenting with high-risk features and a selective invasive approach in low- to intermediate-risk women who are biomarker negative.[44]

## SUMMARY

ACS and STEMI are a major cause of cardiovascular morbidity and mortality in women. However, emerging data now suggest that the poorer outcomes of women undergoing PCI may have less to do with differing vascular biology between males and females or the technical challenges of their coronary anatomy, but more with risk factors, such as age and comorbidities.[9,16] Nevertheless, females have clearly been underrepresented in clinical trials, and further efforts are now required to properly define effective ways to tackle the risk-factor burden and clinical outcomes in women presenting to the catheterization laboratory.

## REFERENCES

1. Roger VL, Go AS, Lloyd-Jones DM, et al. Heart disease and stroke statistics–2011 update: a report from the American Heart Association. Circulation 2011;123:e18–209.
2. Xu J, Kochanek KD, Murphy S, et al. Deaths: final data for 2007. Hyattsville, MD: National Center for Health Statistics. Natl Vital Stat Rep 2010;58:1–135.
3. Biswas MS, Calhoun PS, Bosworth HB, et al. Are women worrying about heart disease? Womens Health Issues 2002;12:204–11.
4. Mosca L, Linfante AH, Benjamin EJ, et al. National study of physician awareness and adherence to cardiovascular disease prevention guidelines. Circulation 2005;111:499–510.

5. Kushner FG, Hand M, Smith SC Jr, et al. 2009 focused updates: ACC/AHA guidelines for the management of patients with ST-elevation myocardial infarction (updating the 2004 guideline and 2007 focused update) and ACC/AHA/SCAI guidelines on percutaneous coronary intervention (updating the 2005 guideline and 2007 focused update) a report of the American College of Cardiology Foundation/ American Heart Association Task Force on Practice Guidelines. J Am Coll Cardiol 2009;54:2205–41.

6. Van de Werf F, Bax J, Betriu A, et al. ESC Committee for Practice Guidelines (CPG). Management of acute myocardial infarction in patients presenting with persistent ST-segment elevation: the Task Force on the Management of ST-Segment Elevation Acute Myocardial Infarction of the European Society of Cardiology. Eur Heart J 2008;29:2909–45.

7. Wright RS, Anderson JL, Adams CD, et al. 2011 ACCF/AHA focused update of the Guidelines for the Management of Patients with Unstable Angina/ Non-ST-Elevation Myocardial Infarction (updating the 2007 guideline): a report of the American College of Cardiology Foundation/American Heart Association Task Force on Practice Guidelines developed in collaboration with the American College of Emergency Physicians, Society for Cardiovascular Angiography and Interventions, and Society of Thoracic Surgeons. J Am Coll Cardiol 2011;57:1920–59.

8. Hamm CW, Bassand JP, Agewall S, et al. ESC Guidelines for the management of acute coronary syndromes in patients presenting without persistent ST-segment elevation: The Task Force for the management of acute coronary syndromes (ACS) in patients presenting without persistent ST-segment elevation of the European Society of Cardiology (ESC). Eur Heart J 2011;32:2999–3054.

9. Kovacic JC, Mehran R, Karajgikar R, et al. Female gender and mortality after percutaneous coronary intervention: results from a large registry. Catheter Cardiovasc Interv 2011. DOI:10.1002/c/cd.23338. [Epub ahead of print].

10. Grady D, Chaput L, Kristof M. Results of systematic review of research on diagnosis and treatment of coronary heart disease in women. Evidence Report/ Technology Assessment No. 80. AHRQ Publication No. 03-0035. Rockville (MD): Agency for Healthcare Research and Quality; 2003.

11. Lansky AJ, Hochman JS, Ward PA, et al. American College of Cardiology Foundation; American Heart Association. Percutaneous coronary intervention and adjunctive pharmacotherapy in women: a statement for healthcare professionals from the American Heart Association. Circulation 2005;111:940–53.

12. Jacobs AK. Coronary intervention in 2009: are women no different than men? Circ Cardiovasc Interv 2009;2:69–78.

13. Mueller C, Neumann FJ, Roskamm H, et al. Women do have an improved long-term outcome after non-ST-elevation acute coronary syndromes treated very early and predominantly with percutaneous coronary intervention: a prospective study in 1,450 consecutive patients. J Am Coll Cardiol 2002;40: 245–50.

14. Vaccarino V, Parsons L, Every NR, et al. Sex-based differences in early mortality after myocardial infarction. National Registry of Myocardial Infarction 2 Participants. N Engl J Med 1999;341:217–25.

15. Bairey Merz CN, Shaw LJ, Reis SE, et al. WISE Investigators. Insights from the NHLBI-Sponsored Women's Ischemia Syndrome Evaluation (WISE) Study: Part II: gender differences in presentation, diagnosis, and outcome with regard to gender-based pathophysiology of atherosclerosis and macrovascular and microvascular coronary disease. J Am Coll Cardiol 2006;47(Suppl 3):S21–9.

16. Kovacic JC, Kini AS. Inferior outcomes in percutaneous coronary interventions: narrowing the gap between men and women. Interv Cardiol 2011;3: 119–21.

17. Roe MT, Parsons LS, Pollack CV Jr, et al; National Registry of Myocardial Infarction Investigators. Quality of care by classification of myocardial infarction: treatment patterns for ST-segment elevation vs non-ST-segment elevation myocardial infarction. Arch Intern Med 2005;165:1630–6.

18. Yeh RW, Sidney S, Chandra M, et al. Population trends in the incidence and outcomes of acute myocardial infarction. N Engl J Med 2010;362: 2155–65.

19. Jneid H, Fonarow GC, Cannon CP, et al. Get With the Guidelines Steering Committee and Investigators. Sex differences in medical care and early death after acute myocardial infarction. Circulation 2008; 118:2803–10.

20. Aylward P, Topol EJ, Califf RM. Sex, clinical presentation, and outcome in patients with acute coronary syndromes. Global Use of Strategies to Open Occluded Coronary Arteries in Acute Coronary Syndromes IIb Investigators. N Engl J Med 1999; 341:226–32.

21. Stone GW, Grines CL, Browne KF, et al. Comparison of in-hospital outcome in men versus women treated by either thrombolytic therapy or primary coronary angioplasty for acute myocardial infarction. Am J Cardiol 1995;75:987–92.

22. White HD, Barbash GI, Modan M, et al. After correcting for worse baseline characteristics, women treated with thrombolytic therapy for acute myocardial infarction have the same mortality and morbidity as men except for a higher incidence of hemorrhagic stroke. The Investigators of the International Tissue Plasminogen Activator/Streptokinase Mortality Study. Circulation 1993;88:2097–103.

23. Woodfield SL, Lundergan CF, Reiner JS, et al. Gender and acute myocardial infarction: is there a different response to thrombolysis? J Am Coll Cardiol 1997;29:35–42.

24. Tamis-Holland JE, Palazzo A, Stebbins AL, et al. GUSTO II-B Angioplasty Substudy Investigators. Benefits of direct angioplasty for women and men with acute myocardial infarction: results of the Global Use of Strategies to Open Occluded Arteries in Acute Coronary Syndromes Angioplasty (GUSTO II-B) Angioplasty Substudy. Am Heart J 2004;147:133–9.

25. Lansky AJ, Pietras C, Costa RA, et al. Gender differences in outcomes after primary angioplasty versus primary stenting with and without abciximab for acute myocardial infarction: results of the Controlled Abciximab and Device Investigation to Lower Late Angioplasty Complications (CADILLAC) trial. Circulation 2005;111:1611–8.

26. Furman MI, Dauerman HL, Goldberg RJ, et al. Twenty-two year (1975 to 1997) trends in the incidence, in-hospital and long-term case fatality rates from initial Q-wave and non-Q-wave myocardial infarction: a multi-hospital, community-wide perspective. J Am Coll Cardiol 2001;37:1571–80.

27. The TIMI IIIB Investigators. Effects of tissue plasminogen activator and a comparison of early invasive and conservative strategies in unstable angina and non-Q-wave myocardial infarction. Results of the TIMI IIIB Trial. Thrombolysis in Myocardial Ischemia. Circulation 1994;89:1545–56.

28. Boden WE, O'Rourke RA, Crawford MH, et al. Outcomes in patients with acute non-Q-wave myocardial infarction randomly assigned to an invasive as compared with a conservative management strategy. Veterans Affairs Non-Q-Wave Infarction Strategies in Hospital (VANQWISH) Trial Investigators. N Engl J Med 1998;338:1785–92.

29. FRagmin and Fast Revascularisation during InStability in Coronary artery disease Investigators. Invasive compared with non-invasive treatment in unstable coronary-artery disease: FRISC II prospective randomised multicentre study. Lancet 1999;354:708–15.

30. Fox KA, Poole-Wilson PA, Henderson RA, et al. Randomized Intervention Trial of unstable Angina Investigators. Interventional versus conservative treatment for patients with unstable angina or non-ST-elevation myocardial infarction: the British Heart Foundation RITA 3 randomised trial. Randomized Intervention Trial of unstable Angina. Lancet 2002;360:743–51.

31. Cannon CP, Weintraub WS, Demopoulos LA, et al. TACTICS (Treat Angina with Aggrastat and Determine Cost of Therapy with an Invasive or Conservative Strategy) -Thrombolysis in Myocardial Infarction 18 Investigators. Comparison of early invasive and conservative strategies in patients with unstable coronary syndromes treated with the glycoprotein IIb/IIIa inhibitor tirofiban. N Engl J Med 2001;344:1879–87.

32. Spacek R, Widimský P, Straka Z, et al. Value of first day angiography/angioplasty in evolving Non-ST segment elevation myocardial infarction: an open multicenter randomized trial. The VINO Study. Eur Heart J 2002;23:230–8.

33. de Winter RJ, Windhausen F, Cornel JH, et al. Invasive versus Conservative Treatment in Unstable Coronary Syndromes (ICTUS) Investigators. Early invasive versus selectively invasive management for acute coronary syndromes. N Engl J Med 2005;353:1095–104.

34. Swahn E, Alfredsson J, Afzal R, et al. Early invasive compared with a selective invasive strategy in women with non-ST-elevation acute coronary syndromes: a substudy of the OASIS 5 trial and a meta-analysis of previous randomized trials. Eur Heart J 2012;33(1):51–60.

35. Lagerqvist B, Säfström K, Ståhle E, et al. FRISC II Study Group Investigators. Is early invasive treatment of unstable coronary artery disease equally effective for both women and men? FRISC II Study Group Investigators. J Am Coll Cardiol 2001;38:41–8.

36. Clayton TC, Pocock SJ, Henderson RA, et al. Do men benefit more than women from an interventional strategy in patients with unstable angina or non-ST-elevation myocardial infarction? The impact of gender in the RITA 3 trial. Eur Heart J 2004;25:1641–50.

37. Glasser R, Herrmann HC, Murphy SA, et al. Benefit of an early invasive management strategy in women with acute coronary syndromes. JAMA 2002;288:3124–9.

38. Mehta SR, Granger CB, Boden WE, et al. TIMACS Investigators. Early versus delayed invasive intervention in acute coronary syndromes. N Engl J Med 2009;360:2165–75.

39. O'Donoghue M, Boden WE, Braunwald E, et al. Early invasive vs conservative treatment strategies in women and men with unstable angina and non-ST-segment elevation myocardial infarction: a meta-analysis. JAMA 2008;300:71–80.

40. Hoenig MR, Aroney CN, Scott IA. Early invasive versus conservative strategies for unstable angina and non-ST elevation myocardial infarction in the stent era. Cochrane Database Syst Rev 2010;3:CD004815.

41. Fox KA, Clayton TC, Damman P, et al. FIR Collaboration. Long-term outcome of a routine versus selective invasive strategy in patients with non-ST-segment elevation acute coronary syndrome a meta-analysis of individual patient data. J Am Coll Cardiol 2010;55:2435–45.

42. Blomkalns AL, Chen AY, Hochman JS, et al. CRUSADE Investigators. Gender disparities in the

diagnosis and treatment of non-ST-segment elevation acute coronary syndromes: large-scale observations from the CRUSADE (Can Rapid Risk
Stratification of Unstable Angina Patients Suppress
Adverse Outcomes With Early Implementation of
the American College of Cardiology/American Heart
Association Guidelines) National Quality Improvement Initiative. J Am Coll Cardiol 2005;45:832–7.

43. Diercks DB, Owen KP, Kontos MC, et al. Gender differences in time to presentation for myocardial infarction
before and after a national women's cardiovascular
awareness campaign: a temporal analysis from the
Can Rapid Risk Stratification of Unstable Angina
Patients Suppress ADverse Outcomes with Early Implementation (CRUSADE) and the National Cardiovascular Data Registry Acute Coronary Treatment
and Intervention Outcomes Network-Get with the
Guidelines (NCDR ACTION Registry-GWTG). Am
Heart J 2010;160:80–7.

44. Anderson JL, Adams CD, Antman EM, et al. American
College of Cardiology/American Heart Association
Task Force on Practice Guidelines (Writing Committee
to Revise the 2002 Guidelines for the Management of
Patients With Unstable Angina/Non-ST-Elevation
Myocardial Infarction), American College of Emergency Physicians, Society for Cardiovascular Angi-
ography and Interventions, Society of Thoracic
Surgeons, American Association of Cardiovascular
and Pulmonary Rehabilitation, Society for Academic
Emergency Medicine. ACC/AHA 2007 guidelines for
the management of patients with unstable angina/
non-ST-Elevation myocardial infarction: a report of
the American College of Cardiology/American Heart
Association Task Force on Practice Guidelines
(Writing Committee to Revise the 2002 Guidelines
for the Management of Patients With Unstable
Angina/Non-ST-Elevation Myocardial Infarction)
developed in collaboration with the American College
of Emergency Physicians, the Society for Cardiovascular Angiography and Interventions, and the Society
of Thoracic Surgeons endorsed by the American
Association of Cardiovascular and Pulmonary Rehabilitation and the Society for Academic Emergency
Medicine. J Am Coll Cardiol 2007;50:e1–157.

# The Generations of Drug-Eluting Stents and Outcomes in Women

Vivian G. Ng, MD[a], Alexandra J. Lansky, MD[b],*

## KEYWORDS

- Drug-eluting stent • Percutaneous coronary intervention
- Women • Gender

Coronary artery disease (CAD) is the leading cause of mortality in both men and women.[1] Over the last several decades, there have been great improvements in revascularization technology in interventional cardiology. Although percutaneous coronary interventions (PCI) have become a mainstay of therapy in acute coronary syndrome (ACS) and ST-segment elevation myocardial infarction (STEMI), women continue to be undertreated with these interventions.[1] In 2007, only approximately 33% of PCI procedures were performed in women.[1] Despite the high prevalence of CAD in women, the prevalence of obstructive CAD is lower[2] and, consequently, women constitute a minority of patients included in trials studying drug-eluting stents (DES). Thus, data assessing the outcomes of women who undergo DES placement are limited. This article reviews the evolution of DES, current DES approved by the Food and Drug Administration, and the impact of these therapies on outcomes in women. The key points of this article are listed in **Box 1**. A summary of outcomes from major DES clinical trials according to gender is provided in **Tables 1** and **2**.

## DEVELOPMENT OF CORONARY STENTING

Coronary artery stents were initially developed to provide a mechanical solution to the acute recoil and abrupt closure observed with standard balloon angioplasty.[3,4] The scaffolding afforded by the original bare metal stents (BMS) provided additional acute luminal gains that translated into reduced restenosis and revascularization rates.[4–6]

## FIRST GENERATION OF DES

Despite the improved acute clinical outcomes achieved with BMS implantation, restenosis rates remained significant in 20% to 30% of cases and higher in more complex patient and lesion subsets, leading to a new therapeutic challenge of highly fibrotic neointimal hyperplasia and in-stent restenosis that was difficult to treat.[7–10] Hence, DES were developed in an attempt to locally deliver potent antiproliferative agents targeting neointimal hyperplasia while retaining the fundamental mechanical scaffold of the stent platform.

### Sirolimus-Eluting Stent

The first-generation Cypher stent comprised 3 components: a stainless-steel stent platform and a durable polymer coating embedded with the antiproliferative agent sirolimus. Sirolimus, an mTOR inhibitor, was selected for its inhibition of smooth muscle cell proliferation and neointimal hyperplasia.[11–13] In clinical trials, the Cypher sirolimus-eluting stent (SES) improved clinical outcomes and decreased rates of restenosis.[14–19]

Disclosures: The authors have nothing to disclose.
[a] Columbia University Medical Center, Medical Housestaff Office, 177 Fort Washington Avenue, 6th Floor, Room 12, New York, NY 10032, USA
[b] Yale University School of Medicine, PO Box 208017, New Haven, CT 06520-8017, USA
* Corresponding author.
E-mail address: alexandra.lansky@yale.edu

Intervent Cardiol Clin 1 (2012) 183–195
doi:10.1016/j.iccl.2012.01.002
2211-7458/12/$ – see front matter © 2012 Elsevier Inc. All rights reserved.

---

**Box 1**
**Key points**

- Drug-eluting stent technology has evolved with refinements in stent platform, polymer coating, and antiproliferative drugs

- Advances in drug-eluting stents have led to improved safety and effective outcomes

- Gender analyses of clinical trials studying outcomes after drug-eluting stent implantation have shown that women have worse risk profiles and outcomes compared with men

- Improvements in drug-eluting stent technology have improved outcomes in women with coronary artery disease

---

The original Randomized Study with the Sirolimus-Coated Bx Velocity Balloon Expandable Stent in the Treatment of Patients with De-Novo Native Coronary Artery Lesions (RAVEL) study randomized 238 patients with low-risk lesions to either a Cypher SES or a BMS stent. This study established proof of concept, demonstrating that binary restenosis rates were significantly reduced with the Cypher SES drug-device combination compared with patients who received the BMS at 1-year follow-up (0.0% vs 26.6%, P<.001).[14] The results were confirmed in the larger, pivotal United States Sirolimus-Eluting Stent in De-Novo Native Coronary Lesions (SIRIUS) trial of 1058 patients.[15] Sustained benefit was established in the SIRIUS trial at 2 years and 5 years,[16,17] and these results have been confirmed in numerous real-world registries.[20–24]

To evaluate the impact of gender on outcomes after SES, a patient-level pooled analysis of 4 trials including RAVEL, SIRIUS, E-SIRIUS (sirolimus-eluting stents for treatment of patients with long atherosclerotic lesions in small coronary arteries), and C-SIRIUS (Canadian study of the sirolimus-eluting stent in the treatment of patients with long de novo lesions in small native coronary arteries) was performed.[25] A total of 1748 patients (497 [28.4%] women) were included in this analysis. Although women had worse baseline risk profiles, they had similar outcomes compared with men when treated with SES. Women who were treated with SES rather than BMS had lower rates of in-segment binary restenosis (6.3% vs 43.8%, P<.0001). Furthermore, rates of major adverse cardiac events (8.1% vs 22.3%, P<.0001), myocardial infarction (MI; 2.4% vs 16.1%, P = .04), target lesion revascularization (4.1% vs 18.3%, P<.0001) and target vessel revascularization (6.9% vs 20.4%, P<.0001) were

significantly lower in women randomized to SES compared with those treated with BMS. Women had similar outcomes compared with men after PCI up to 1 year and, more importantly, women had improved outcomes after SES implantation in comparison with women treated with BMS implantation. However, it is unclear whether long-term outcomes with SES are similar between men and women. A retrospective study containing 1186 patients (216 [18.2%] women) who were treated with SES found that women had higher rates than men of target vessel revascularization (3.9% vs 0.95, P = .001) after a median follow-up period of 33.2 months.[26] Whether women are more prone to a late catch-up phenomenon is not clear, and a long-term analysis of outcomes in women treated with and without SES has not been performed.

## Paclitaxel-Eluting Stent

The other first-generation DES, the TAXUS paclitaxel-eluting stent (PES), is a stainless-steel stent platform with a durable polymer coating that elutes paclitaxel. Paclitaxel inhibits microtubule function and arrests the mitotic cell cycle. Studies found that patients receiving the TAXUS PES had superior outcomes to patients who received a BMS.[18,27–33] The TAXUS-IV trial randomized 1314 patients to stent implantation with TAXUS PES or a BMS. At 9-month follow-up, patients who received the TAXUS PES had lower rates of target vessel revascularization (4.7% vs 12.0%, P<.001) and target lesion revascularization (3.0% vs 11.3%, P<.001) compared with patients treated with a BMS,[29] with sustained reductions in target vessel revascularization (16.9% vs 27.4%, P<.0001) and target lesion revascularization (9.1% vs 20.5%, P<.0001) at 5 years.[31] In addition, the Taxus Stent Evaluated at Rotterdam Cardiology Hospital (T-SEARCH) registry found that the TAXUS PES had similar efficacy in reducing restenosis in comparison with the Cypher SES in a real-world registry.[34,35]

A gender subanalysis of the TAXUS-IV trial demonstrated that women benefited from TAXUS Express PES use compared with BMS use.[36] This trial consisted of 367 women (187 randomized to PES, 180 randomized to BMS). Women were older than men and in comparison had more hypertension, diabetes, and renal insufficiency. Women who received the TAXUS stent had higher rates of target lesion revascularization (7.6% vs 3.2%, P = .03) compared with men, despite similar rates of restenosis (8.6% vs 7.6%, P = .80) at 1 year. In a multivariate analysis, female gender was not an independent predictor of target lesion

**Table 1**
Summary of outcomes after drug-eluting stent implantation: studies comparing men and women

| Authors[Ref.] | Study Name | Treatment | No. of Patients | Length of Follow-Up | Outcome (%) |
|---|---|---|---|---|---|
| **Randomized Controlled Trials** | | | | | |
| Solinas et al[25] | RAVEL, SIRIUS, E-SIRIUS, C-SIRIUS | SES | 629 men vs 249 women | 1 y | BR: 6.4 vs 6.3, $P$ = 1.00<br>MACE: 7.7 vs 8.1, $P$ = .87<br>MI: 3.7 vs 2.45, $P$ = .34<br>TLR: 4.3 vs 4.1, $P$ = .86 |
| Lansky et al[36] | TAXUS IV | PES | 947 men vs 367 women | 9 mo<br>1 y | BR: 8.6 vs 7.6, $P$ = .80<br>MACE: 9.9 vs 13.5, $P$ = .24<br>TLR: 3.2 vs 7.6, $P$ = .03<br>TVR: 5.7 vs 10.8, $P$ = .03 |
| Mikhail et al[40] | TAXUS I, II, IV, V, ATLAS | PES | 1606 men vs 665 women | 5 y | Death: 1.71 vs 1.69, $P$ = .97<br>TLR: 2.67 vs 2.85, $P$ = .67 |
| Brown et al[52] | ENDEAVOR I–IV | ZES | 1524 men vs 608 women | 8 mo<br>2 y | BR: 13.9 vs 10.4, $P$ = .18<br>MACE: 10.2 vs 8.8, $P$ = .01<br>TVR: 11.9 vs 10.1, $P$ = .005 |
| Lansky et al[66] | SPIRIT III | EES and PES | 687 men vs 314 women | 1 y | MACE: 5.7 vs 11.1, $P$ = .0036<br>TVF: 7.5 vs 13.7, $P$ = .003 |
| Ng et al[67] | SPIRIT III | EES and PES | 687 men vs 314 women | 3 y | MACE: 5.7 vs 11.1, $P$ = .0036<br>TVF: 7.5 vs 13.7, $P$ = .003 |
| Seth et al[68] | SPIRIT II and III | EES and PES | 906 men vs 395 women | 2 y | MACE: 7.9 vs 11.1, $P$ = .05<br>TVF: 11.2 vs 13.9, $P$ = .1 |
| **Registry Studies** | | | | | |
| Trabbatoni et al[26] | | SES | 970 men vs 216 women | Median 33.2 mo | Cardiac death: 0.4 vs 0, $P$ = NS<br>TVR: 0.9 vs 3.9, $P$ = .001 |
| Mikhail et al[40] | ARRIVE 1 and 2 | PES | Simple use: 1777 men vs 921 women<br>Expanded use: 3266 men vs 1528 women | 2 y<br>2 y | Death: 2.07 vs 2.34, $P$ = .55<br>TLR: 2.60 vs 3.27, $P$ = .19<br>Death: 3.74 vs 4.82, $P$ = .02<br>TLR 4.60 vs 5.82, $P$ = .02 |
| Abbott et al[41] | NHLBI Registry | SES and PES | 1132 men vs 631 women | 1 y | MACE: 15.6 vs 15.7, $P$ = .98<br>Death: 3.6 vs 3.8, $P$ = .97 |
| Onuma et al[43] | RESEARCH and T-SEARCH | SES and PES | 2007 men vs 798 women | 3 y | MACE: 19.1 vs 20.9, $P$ = .027<br>Death: 9.5 vs 10.2, $P$ = .52<br>TVR: 9.7 vs 10.3, $P$ = .72 |
| Danzi et al[81] | Nobori | Nobori stent | 806 men vs 194 women | 6 mo | MACE: 3.1 vs 4.3, $P$ = NS |

*Abbreviations:* BMS, bare metal stent; BR, binary restenosis; DES, drug-eluting stent; EES, everolimus-eluting stent; MACE, major adverse cardiac events; MI, myocardial infarction; NS, not significant; PES, paclitaxel-eluting stent; TLR, target lesions revascularization; TVF, target vessel failure; TVR, target vessel revascularization; ZES, zotarolimus-eluting stent.

**Table 2**
Summary of outcomes after drug-eluting stent implantation in women

| Authors[Ref.] | Study Name | Treatment | No. of Patients | Length of Follow-Up | Outcome (%) |
|---|---|---|---|---|---|
| Randomized Controlled Trials | | | | | |
| Solinas et al[25] | RAVEL, SIRIUS, E-SIRIUS, C-SIRIUS | SES vs BMS | 249 SES vs 248 BMS | 1 y | BR: 6.3 vs 43.8, $P<.0001$<br>MACE: 8.1 vs 22.3, $P<.0001$<br>MI: 2.4 vs 16.1, $P = .04$<br>TLR: 4.1 vs 18.3, $P<.001$ |
| Lansky et al[36] | TAXUS IV | PES vs BMS | 187 PES vs 180 BMS | 9 mo<br>1 y | BR: 8.6 vs 29.2, $P = .0001$<br>MACE: 13.5 vs 19.0, $P = .02$<br>TLR: 7.6 vs14.9, $P = .02$<br>TVR: 10.8 vs 17.5, $P = .07$ |
| Mikhail et al[40] | TAXUS I, II, IV, V, ATLAS | PES vs BMS | 665 PES vs 395 BMS | 5 y | TLR: 11.5 vs 22.6, $P<.001$ |
| Brown et al[52] | ENDEAVOR I–IV | ZES vs BMS | 608 ZES vs 147 BMS | 8 mo<br>2 y | BR: 10.4 vs 36.8, $P<.001$<br>MACE: 8.8 vs 20.1, $P = .0002$<br>TVR: 10.1 vs 18.8, $P = .001$ |
| Lansky et al[66] | SPIRIT III | EES vs PES | 200 EES vs 114 PES | 1 y | MACE: 8.2 vs 16.1, $P = .04$<br>TVF: 11.3 vs 17.9, $P = .12$ |
| Ng et al[67] | SPIRIT III | EES vs PES | 200 EES vs 114 PES | 3 y | MACE: 12.2 vs 22.6, $P = .033$<br>TVF: 16.0 vs 26.4, $P = .03$ |
| Seth et al[68] | SPIRIT II and III | EES vs PES | 265 EES vs 130 PES | 2 y | MACE: 8.5 vs 16.4, $P = .002$<br>TVF: 11.2 vs 19.5, $P = .02$ |
| Windecker[69] | SPIRIT Women | EES vs SES | 304 EES vs 151 SES | 1 y | MACE: 18.8 vs 18.7, $P = 1.00$<br>Death: 1.4 vs 4.0, $P = .09$ |
| Registry Studies | | | | | |
| Onuma et al[43] | RESEARCH and T-SEARCH | SES and PES vs BMS | 798 DES vs 596 BMS | 3 y | MACE: 19.1 vs 25.9, $P = .03$<br>Death: 9.5 vs 11.6, $P = .44$<br>TVR: 10.3 vs 14.7, $P = .02$ |
| Kedhi et al[65] | COMPARE | EES vs PES | 278 EES vs 249 PES | 1 y | MACE 6 vs 11, $P = .07$ |

*Abbreviations:* BMS, bare metal stent; BR, binary restenosis; DES, drug-eluting stent; EES, everolimus-eluting stent; MACE, major adverse cardiac events; MI, myocardial infarction; PES, paclitaxel-eluting stent; TLR, target lesions revascularization; TVR, target vessel revascularization; TVF, target vessel failure; ZES, zotarolimus-eluting stent.

revascularization. Among women, treatment with the TAXUS stent was associated with less restenosis at 9 months (8.6% vs 29.2%, $P = .0001$) and lower rates of target lesion revascularization (7.6% vs 14.9%, $P = .02$). Both men and women had an approximately 70% reduction of angiographic restenosis, and randomization to the TAXUS stent was an independent predictor of freedom from restenosis in women (odds ratio 0.28 [0.11, 0.74], $P = .01$). Thus, although women had worse outcomes than men in this trial, treatment with the TAXUS stent instead of a BMS resulted in improved outcomes in women.

The TAXUS PES underwent further modifications to improve device performance and delivery. The TAXUS Liberté stent used a stainless-steel platform with thinner stent struts to improve deliverability and afford a more uniform cell geometry, to provide a more homogeneous support and distribution of paclitaxel to the vessel wall. The design of the TAXUS Liberté stent varies with stent diameter, such that stents with a diameter between 2.25 and 2.5 mm have a 2-cell stent design, and stents with a diameter of more than 2.75 mm have a 3-cell stent design.[37] The TAXUS Liberté-SR Stent for the Treatment of De Novo Coronary Artery Lesion (TAXUS ATLAS) multicenter clinical trial demonstrated that the TAXUS Liberté stent was noninferior to the TAXUS Express PES, with similar rates of 9-month target vessel revascularization (7.95% vs 7.01%, $P = .049$).[37] The TAXUS ATLAS Small Vessels study demonstrated noninferiority to the TAXUS Express PES in small vessels, with significantly lower 9-month angiographic restenosis with the TAXUS Liberté (18.5% vs 32.7%, $P = .02$) and lower rates of target lesion revascularization at 1 year (6.1% vs 16.9%, $P = .004$).[38] Results in small vessels were sustained at 3-year follow-up with the TAXUS Liberté in comparison with TAXUS Express (TLR: 10.0% vs 22.1%, $P = .008$).[39] This information is particularly important for the treatment of women, because women are more likely to have small vessels and thus would benefit from the improved size-dependent PES design. However, a gender analysis of the TAXUS Liberté stent has not been performed.

The long-term benefits of PES (TAXUS Express stent and TAXUS Liberté stent) in women were assessed in the TAXUS Women analysis, a pooled analysis of 5 randomized clinical trials (TAXUS I, II, IV, V, ATLAS) and 2 real-world registries (TAXUS Peri-Approved Registry: A Multicenter Safety Surveillance [ARRIVE] 1 and 2).[40] Among the 2271 patients (665 [29.3%] women) from the 5 randomized trials, women had higher risk profiles than men; however, they had similar long-term

outcomes compared with men. Women who received PES had lower rates of target lesion revascularization than women who received a BMS through the 5-year follow-up period (11.5% vs 22.6%, $P<.001$). The registry patients were divided into those who underwent stenting for simple use and those who received stenting for expanded use. Although women and men had similar outcomes in the simple-use group, women had higher rates of target lesion revascularization in the expanded-use group at 2-year follow-up compared with men (5.82% vs 4.60%, $P = .02$). Thus, these data suggest that both men and women have improved long-term outcomes when receiving PES rather than BMS; however, in the real-world setting, women may have worse outcomes than men when PES is used for off-label purposes.

The overall benefits of both first-generation stents (SES and PES) in women have been confirmed in large registry studies that contained patients with more severe and complex disease than the patients in the randomized trials.[41-43] Using the National Heart, Lung and Blood Institute Dynamic Registry, outcomes of 4159 patients who received either a BMS (631 women, 1132 men) or DES (486 women, 974 men) between October 2001 and May 2004 were compared according to treatment and gender.[41] In both the DES and BMS groups, women were older and had higher rates of diabetes, hypertension, and congestive heart failure than men, and had smaller reference vessel diameters. Compared with men, women had higher rates of bleeding requiring a transfusion, whether they received a BMS (3.0% vs 0.8%, $P<.001$) or a DES (3.5% vs 0.2%, $P<.001$). However, there were no differences in the rates of major adverse cardiovascular events, death, MI, or stent thrombosis at 1-year follow-up between men and women. Among women, those who had received a DES had a lower rate of clinically driven repeat PCI compared with women who received a BMS at 1 year (14.1% vs 9.5%, $P = .02$). By multivariable analysis, DES implantation was associated with a lower risk of repeat revascularization in women (relative risk 0.61 [0.41, 0.89], $P = .01$). Furthermore, a study combining patients from the RESEARCH and T-SEARCH registries found that treatment with DES (SES or PES) was associated with lower rates of 3-year target vessel revascularization (hazard ratio 0.52 [0.36, 0.75]) and major adverse cardiac events (hazard ratio 0.63 [0.48, 0.83]) in women.[43] Thus, compared with women who receive a BMS, women who receive either SES or PES have improved clinical outcomes in both short-term and long-term follow-up in real-world practice.

## SECOND GENERATION OF DES

In efforts to further improve the safety and efficacy of DES, second-generation devices have focused on achieving platforms with thinner stent struts, reduced polymer thickness, and more potent antiproliferative agents. Cobalt chromium has characteristics that allow thinner stent struts while maintaining optimal radial strength, and its density retains radiopacity on angiography. Thus the profile the cobalt chrome stent is lower, allowing improved deliverability to the target site even in complex lesions, and may decrease the stimulus for neointimal hyperplasia leading to restenosis.[44,45] In addition, thinner struts may decrease the risk of jailed side-branch occlusions, which can lead to periprocedural myonecrosis.[46]

### Zotarolimus-Eluting Stent

The Endeavor zotarolimus-eluting stent (ZES) is a second-generation stent with a cobalt chromium stent platform. This stent has thin struts (96.3 μm compared with 152.6 μm in SES and 132 μm in PES) coated with a permanent biocompatible phosphorylcholine polymer, which may cause less inflammation than standard poly(lactic acid) polymers. The Endeavor stent has improved outcomes compared with the Driver BMS in the Clinical Evaluation of the Medtronic ACE ABT-578 Coated Driver Coronary Stent in De Novo Native Coronary Artery Lesions (ENDEAVOR) II trial, which randomized 1197 patients to either the Endeavor ZES or a BMS. Patients who received the Endeavor ZES had lower rates of target vessel failure (7.9% vs 15.1%, $P = .0001$) and target lesion revascularization (4.6% vs 11.8%, $P = .0001$) at 9 months.[47–49] In the Endeavor IV trial, which randomized 1548 patients to either ZES or PES, ZES implantation resulted in lower rates of periprocedural MI compared with PES (0.5% vs 2.2%, $P = .0007$), which was thought to be a result of decreased side-branch occlusions in patients treated with ZES.[49] The ZES had a better safety profile than first-generation SES and PES.[50,51] For example, in the 3-year follow-up of the ENDEAVOR IV trial, patients who received a ZES had lower rates of cardiac death/MI (3.6% vs 7.1%, $P = .004$), MI (2.1% vs 4.9%, $P = .005$), target vessel failure (12.3% vs 15.9%, $P = .049$), and very late definite/probable stent thrombosis (0.1% vs 1.4%, $P = .006$).[50]

A pooled meta-analysis of the 6 prospective multicenter ENDEAVOR trials containing 2132 patients (608 [28.5%] women) was performed to determine whether gender had an impact on the outcomes of patients receiving the Endeavor ZES.[52] Among ZES-treated patients, women were older (67.0 [58.0, 74.0] years vs 61.0 [54.0, 69.0] years, $P<.001$) and had higher rates of diabetes (33.7% vs 23.0%, $P<.001$) and hypertension (80.1% vs 70.1%, $P<.001$), and had smaller reference vessel diameters (2.64 [2.34, 2.94] mm vs 2.73 [2.41, 3.07] mm, $P<.001$) than men. At 8-month angiographic follow-up, there were no significant differences between men and women. However, at 2 years, women had lower rates of major adverse cardiovascular events (8.8% vs 10.2%, $P = .01$) and target vessel failure (9.9% vs 12.8%, $P = .0004$) driven by lower rates of clinically driven target vessel revascularization (10.1% vs 11.9%, $P = .005$). Within the female subgroup, women who were treated with ZES had significant reductions in in-stent binary restenosis (8.3% vs 36.8%, $P<.001$) in comparison with women treated with BMS at 8-month angiographic follow-up. At 2-year follow-up, women receiving the ZES had lower rates of target lesion revascularization (7.9% vs 17.4%, $P = .0003$) and target vessel failure (9.9% vs 21.5%, $P = .0003$) than women receiving BMS. There were no differences in death, MI, or stent thrombosis rates between the ZES and BMS female treatment arms. Thus, despite the higher rates of comorbidities in women, this meta-analysis suggests that women have improved clinical outcomes compared with men. It is unclear whether there was a difference in biological response to ZES between men and women, or whether there was a treatment bias. Although women and men had similar rates and extent of restenosis, women had lower rates of repeat revascularization, suggesting that there may have been a higher threshold in a female patient than in a male patient before clinicians intervened on a lesion. Of importance, women treated with ZES had improved clinical outcomes compared with women treated with BMS, without an increase in stent thrombosis. However, a study comparing the outcomes of ZES implantation with the outcomes of first-generation DES in women has not been performed.

The Resolute stent has the same thin strut design and zotarolimus drug as the Endeavor ZES, but prolongs the delivery of zotarolimus over time by using BioLinx tripolymer coating, a 3-polymer blend coating, to match the delayed endothelial healing found in complex lesions.[53,54] The multicenter Resolute All Comer noninferiority trial, with few exclusion criteria, randomized 2292 patients to either the Resolute stent or the Xience V stent, and demonstrated that the Resolute ZES had noninferior rates of target lesion failure at 1 year (8.2% vs 8.3%, $P<.001$) and extent of in-stent stenosis (21.65% ± 14.42% vs 19.76%

± 14.64%) at 13 months compared with the Xience V stent,[55] with similar clinical and angiographic outcomes up to 2 years.[56] Furthermore, the RESOLUTE US trial, comparing 1402 patients receiving the Resolute ZES to historical Endeavor ZES patient data from the ENDEAVOR trials, demonstrated that target lesion failure after Resolute ZES implantation is noninferior to Endeavor ZES at 1 year (3.7% vs 6.5%, $P<.001$).[57] Thus, Resolute ZES is an effective therapy in the treatment of both simple and complex lesions. A gender analysis has not been performed for the Resolute ZES at this time.

## Everolimus-Eluting Stent

The second-generation Xience V everolimus-eluting stent (EES) is another cobalt chromium stent with thin struts (88.6 μm) coated with a biocompatible polymer. Early studies demonstrated efficacy of the Xience V EES compared with BMS and first-generation DES implantation.[58–64] The SPIRIT III Trial, randomizing 1002 patients to either Xience V EES or TAXUS PES, demonstrated lower rates of major adverse cardiac events at 1 year with the Xience V EES compared with the TAXUS PES (6.0% vs 10.3%, $P = .02$),[60] with sustained benefits at 3-year follow-up, lower rates of target vessel failure (13.5% vs 19.2%, $P = .03$), and major adverse cardiac events (9.1% vs 15.7%, $P = .003$).[64] These results were duplicated in the expanded randomized SPIRIT IV[61] and COMPARE trials. COMPARE enrolled 1800 patients (527 [29.3%] women) randomized to either the Xience V EES or the TAXUS Liberté PES. Patients receiving the EES had lower rates of all-cause death/MI/target vessel revascularization (6% vs 9%, $P = .02$), MI (3% vs 5%, $P = .007$), target vessel revascularization (2% vs 6%, $P = .001$), and stent thrombosis (<1% vs 3%, $P = .002$) compared with patients receiving the TAXUS Liberté PES at 1 year.[65]

The benefits observed with Xience V implantation are generalizable to women. A gender analysis of the SPIRIT III trial revealed that women had worse outcomes than men, including higher rates of 1-year major adverse cardiac events (11.1% vs 5.7%, $P = .004$) and target vessel failure (13.7% vs 7.5% $P = .003$), which persisted even after adjustment for baseline clinical and angiographic characteristics. Nonetheless, women who were treated with the Xience V stent had lower in-stent late loss (0.19 vs 0.42 mm, $P = .01$) compared with women who received the TAXUS stent. More importantly, women who were treated with Xience V stents had lower rates of 1-year major adverse cardiac events (8.2% vs 16.1%,

$P = .04$) and target vessel revascularization (3.1% vs 8.9%, $P = .03$) than women who were treated with TAXUS stents.[66] Furthermore, Xience V women continued to have lower major adverse cardiac event rates than TAXUS women at 2 years (9.5% vs 18.3%, $P = .03$) and 3 years (12.2% vs 22.6%, $P = .03$). Stent thrombosis rates were infrequent and similar between the 2 treatment groups.[67] These results are consistent with the 2-year results of a pooled analysis of patients from the SPIRIT II and III trials.[68] Furthermore, in a subgroup analysis of the COMPARE trial, which looked at DES use in a real-world setting, there was a trend for decreased rates of major adverse cardiac events in women treated with EES compared with women treated with PES (6% vs 11%, $P = .07$), and there was no significant gender treatment interaction ($P = .59$).[65]

The Xience V SPIRIT Women study is unique in its evaluation of women. This dedicated, prospective, multicenter registry with a nested single-blind randomized study comparing EES with SES is currently ongoing. The SPIRIT Women trial randomizing 304 women to Xience V and 200 women to Cypher SES demonstrated noninferior in-stent late-loss rates between Xience V and Cypher (0.20 ± 0.38 vs 0.12 ± 0.36, $P<.006$) at 9 months, and similar rates of death/MI/target vessel revascularization (21.5% vs 22.0%, $P = .90$) at 1 year.[69] In the SPIRIT Women prospective, open-label, single-arm, all-comer multicenter study, women had low rates of death/MI/target vessel revascularization (12%), target lesion revascularization (2.4%), and stent thrombosis (0.59%) at 1 year.[70] Thus, the Xience V stent is safe and effective in women.

## NEXT-GENERATION STENTS

Next-generation stents continue to optimize the stent platform with bioengineering feats of balancing thinner stent struts while maintaining radial strength and radiopacity. A shift to biodegradable polymer technologies is the current focus of next-generation stents with the aim of minimizing persistent inflammation resulting from endothelial exposure of durable polymers once the drug is eluted, which subsequently causes delayed healing[71] and, possibly, late and very late stent thrombosis.[72,73]

### New Stent Platform: TAXUS Element Paclitaxel-Eluting Stent

The TAXUS Element PES is a platinum-chromium alloy with a thin stent-strut design (81 μm), with improved radiopacity, radial strength, conformability, and biocompatibility.[74,75] The Prospective

Evaluation in a Randomized Trial of the Safety and Efficacy of the Use of the TAXUS Element Paclitaxel-Eluting Coronary Stent System for the Treatment of De Novo Coronary Artery Lesions (PERSEUS) trial randomized 1262 patients (275 [29.2%] women) to either the TAXUS Element stent or the TAXUS Express stent.[76] Target lesion failure at 1 year was noninferior (5.57% vs 6.14%, Bayesian posterior probability of noninferiority = 0.9996) with the TAXUS Element stent in comparison with the TAXUS Express stent. The PERSEUS Small Vessel study (2.25–2.75 mm reference vessel diameters) demonstrated that compared with historical control BMS, the TAXUS Element stent had significantly less late loss ($0.38 \pm 0.51$ vs $0.80 \pm 0.53$ mm, $P<.001$) and lower rates of target lesion failure (7.3% vs 19.5%, $P<.001$).[77] Women receiving the TAXUS Element PES had significantly less in-stent late loss at 9 months ($0.41 \pm 0.48$ vs $0.80 \pm 0.50$, $P = .0001$) and had a trend toward less target lesion failure (5.0% vs 17.0%, $P = .55$) than women receiving a BMS in the historical control group. There was no gender-treatment interaction for either end point, suggesting generalizability of these results to women.[78]

### Bioresorbable Polymer: Biolimus A9 Eluting Stent

Stents are now being developed with biodegradable polymer coatings; however, these devices are in the early stages of clinical evaluation. Thus far, stents using biolimus A9 with a biodegradable polymer coating, namely the Biomatrix stent and the Nobori stent, have the most published data. The polymer used to coat these stents degrades to water and carbon dioxide in 6 to 9 months. The Biomatrix biolimus A9 eluting stent (BES) was studied in the Limus Eluted from a Durable versus Erodable Stent coating (LEADERS) trial, which contained 1707 patients and compared the Biomatrix BES with the Cypher SES.[79,80] It found that treatment with BES was noninferior to SES treatment of the primary end point (composite of cardiac death, myocardial infarction, and clinically driven target vessel revascularization) at 1 year (10.6% vs 12.0%, hazard ratio 0.88 [0.66,1.17], $P = .37$). Furthermore, rates of cardiac death (2.1% vs 2.7%, hazard ratio 0.77 [0.42, 1.44], $P = .42$), MI (5.8% vs 4.6%, hazard ratio 1.27 [0.84, 1.94], $P = .29$), and definite/probable stent thrombosis (2.7% vs 2.2%, $P = .55$) were similar between BES and SES. No gender analysis has been published to date.

The Nobori stent also uses the biolimus A9 drug delivered via a biodegradable polymer. This stent

was studied in the 243-patient Nobori 1 trial, which randomized patients to either the Nobori BES or the TAXUS Liberté PES. Patients treated with the Nobori BES had less in-stent late loss ($0.11 \pm 0.30$ mm vs $0.32 \pm 0.50$, $P = .001$) and binary restenosis (0.7% vs 6.2%, $P = .02$) at 9 months. Both the Nobori BES and TAXUS PES had low rates of major adverse cardiac events at 9 months (4.6% vs 5.6%). A gender analysis of a 1000-patient subset including 194 (19.4%) women who received the Nobori BES found that women had similarly low rates of major adverse cardiac events as men (4.3% vs 3.1%, $P$ not significant) despite having worse baseline characteristics.[81] This trial offers encouraging results for the Nobori BES.

### Fully Bioresorbable Stents

Current stent technology provides permanent radial support and antiproliferative agents to prevent negative vessel remodeling and smooth muscle proliferation after PCI. However, concerns about stent thrombosis and incomplete endothelial healing remain. Because the need for mechanical scaffolding to the arterial wall is only temporary, there are efforts to create fully bioresorbable stents. Furthermore, fully biodegradable stents offer several advantages over current permanent stents, including avoidance of side-branch occlusions, facilitation of future interventions to the same target site, and elimination of image distortion with computed tomography and magnetic resonance imaging.[82] Current biodegradable stents consist of fully bioresorbable polymers. These technologies have been limited by radiolucency on angiograms making optimal placement difficult, and increased strut thickness and decreased radial strength compared with current stents. Fully bioresorbable stent technology is still undergoing clinical investigations.

The ABSORB (A Bioresorbable Everolimus-Eluting Coronary Stent System for Patients with Single De-Novo Coronary Artery Lesion) cohort A study was a multicenter, prospective, open-label first-in-man study containing 30 patients with de novo CAD who received the ABSORB everolimus-eluting bioresorbable vascular scaffold. This stent, which provides similar initial radial strength to that of the Xience V EES,[83] is composed of poly(lactic acid) and is coated with a matrix of polymer and everolimus. At 6-month follow-up, there was only 1 ischemia-driven major adverse cardiac event (non–Q-wave MI), with no further events occurring between 6 months and 4 years of follow-up, including no stent thrombosis events.[84] In addition, there was full resorption of the stent by 2 years according to intravascular ultrasonography and optical coherence tomography.[85] However, 6-month late loss with the ABSORB stent was higher than rates seen with the Xience V EES.[86] As a result, a second-generation ABSORB stent was developed that prolongs the mechanical strength of the stent, and was shown to have improved late lumen loss at 6 months (0.19 mm)[87] and decreased shrinkage compared with the first-generation ABSORB stent.[88] At 1-year follow-up of the ABSORB cohort B study, the second-generation ABSORB stent had similar late loss (0.27 mm) and major adverse cardiac events rates (7.1%) in comparison with previously reported rates for the Xience V stent.[89] These results are encouraging, and a trial comparing this bioresorbable EES with the current metallic EES is under way.

## SUMMARY

There have been many advances in DES technology by improving the stent platform, and developing antiproliferative agents and new biodegradable polymers. Women comprise a minority of patients in the large clinical trials studying DES outcomes, thus there are limited data on women's outcomes with these stents. Nevertheless, gender subset analyses have demonstrated that although women have worse outcomes than men, women have benefited from the advances in DES as evidenced by lower restenosis and revascularization rates compared with BMS. Comparisons of outcomes between women and men treated with DES frequently have demonstrated worse results in women, due to women's worse risk profile on presentation. Such findings have been misconstrued as providing evidence that DES are ineffective in women.[90] However, DES have consistently demonstrated significant clinical benefit compared with BMS in women. Formal gender subanalyses and gender-treatment interaction testing should be an integral part of all future studies of newer-generation DES.

## REFERENCES

1. Roger VL, Go AS, Lloyd-Jones DM, et al. Heart disease and stroke statistics—2011 update: a report from the American Heart Association. Circulation 2011;123:e18–209.
2. Shaw LJ, Min JK, Narula J, et al. Sex differences in mortality associated with computed tomographic angiographic measurements of obstructive and nonobstructive coronary artery disease: an exploratory analysis. Circ Cardiovasc Imaging 2010;3:473–81.
3. Sigwart U, Puel J, Mirkovitch V, et al. Intravascular stents to prevent occlusion and restenosis after transluminal angioplasty. N Engl J Med 1987;316:701–6.
4. de Feyter PJ, de Jaegere PP, Serruys PW. Incidence, predictors, and management of acute coronary occlusion after coronary angioplasty. Am Heart J 1994;127:643–51.
5. Serruys PW, de Jaegere P, Kiemeneij F, et al. A comparison of balloon-expandable-stent implantation with balloon angioplasty in patients with coronary artery disease. Benestent Study Group. N Engl J Med 1994;331:489–95.
6. Fischman DL, Leon MB, Baim DS, et al. A randomized comparison of coronary-stent placement and balloon angioplasty in the treatment of coronary artery disease. Stent Restenosis Study Investigators. N Engl J Med 1994;331:496–501.
7. Hoffmann R, Mintz GS, Dussaillant GR, et al. Patterns and mechanisms of in-stent restenosis. A serial intravascular ultrasound study. Circulation 1996;94:1247–54.
8. Kastrati A, Elezi S, Dirschinger J, et al. Influence of lesion length on restenosis after coronary stent placement. Am J Cardiol 1999;83:1617–22.
9. Elezi S, Kastrati A, Pache J, et al. Diabetes mellitus and the clinical and angiographic outcome after coronary stent placement. J Am Coll Cardiol 1998;32:1866–73.
10. Akiyama T, Moussa I, Reimers B, et al. Angiographic and clinical outcome following coronary stenting of small vessels: a comparison with coronary stenting of large vessels. J Am Coll Cardiol 1998;32:1610–8.
11. Poon M, Marx SO, Gallo R, et al. Rapamycin inhibits vascular smooth muscle cell migration. J Clin Invest 1996;98:2277–83.
12. Marx SO, Marks AR. Bench to bedside: the development of rapamycin and its application to stent restenosis. Circulation 2001;104:852–5.
13. Gallo R, Padurean A, Jayaraman T, et al. Inhibition of intimal thickening after balloon angioplasty in porcine coronary arteries by targeting regulators of the cell cycle. Circulation 1999;99:2164–70.
14. Morice MC, Serruys PW, Sousa JE, et al. A randomized comparison of a sirolimus-eluting stent with a standard stent for coronary revascularization. N Engl J Med 2002;346:1773–80.
15. Moses JW, Leon MB, Popma JJ, et al. Sirolimus-eluting stents versus standard stents in patients with stenosis in a native coronary artery. N Engl J Med 2003;349:1315–23.
16. Weisz G, Leon MB, Holmes DR Jr, et al. Two-year outcomes after sirolimus-eluting stent implantation: results from the Sirolimus-Eluting Stent in de Novo Native Coronary Lesions (SIRIUS) trial. J Am Coll Cardiol 2006;47:1350–5.
17. Weisz G, Leon MB, Holmes DR Jr, et al. Five-year follow-up after sirolimus-eluting stent implantation results of the SIRIUS (Sirolimus-Eluting Stent in

De-Novo Native Coronary Lesions) Trial. J Am Coll Cardiol 2009;53:1488–97.

18. Stone GW, Moses JW, Ellis SG, et al. Safety and efficacy of sirolimus- and paclitaxel-eluting coronary stents. N Engl J Med 2007;356:998–1008.

19. Kastrati A, Mehilli J, Pache J, et al. Analysis of 14 trials comparing sirolimus-eluting stents with bare-metal stents. N Engl J Med 2007;356:1030–9.

20. Lemos PA, Serruys PW, van Domburg RT, et al. Unrestricted utilization of sirolimus-eluting stents compared with conventional bare stent implantation in the "real world": the Rapamycin-Eluting Stent Evaluated At Rotterdam Cardiology Hospital (RESEARCH) registry. Circulation 2004;109:190–5.

21. Daemen J, Kukreja N, van Twisk PH, et al. Four-year clinical follow-up of the rapamycin-eluting stent evaluated at Rotterdam Cardiology Hospital registry. Am J Cardiol 2008;101:1105–11.

22. Serruys PW, Ong AT, Morice MC, et al. Arterial Revascularisation Therapies Study Part II—sirolimus-eluting stents for the treatment of patients with multivessel de novo coronary artery lesions. EuroIntervention 2005;1:147–56.

23. Serruys PW, Daemen J, Morice MC, et al. Three-year follow-up of the ARTS-II—sirolimus-eluting stents for the treatment of patients with multivessel coronary artery disease. EuroIntervention 2008;3:450–9.

24. Serruys PW, Onuma Y, Garg S, et al. 5-year clinical outcomes of the ARTS II (Arterial Revascularization Therapies Study II) of the sirolimus-eluting stent in the treatment of patients with multivessel de novo coronary artery lesions. J Am Coll Cardiol 2010;55:1093–101.

25. Solinas E, Nikolsky E, Lansky AJ, et al. Gender-specific outcomes after sirolimus-eluting stent implantation. J Am Coll Cardiol 2007;50:2111–6.

26. Trabattoni D, Fabbiocchi F, Galli S, et al. Sex difference in long-term clinical outcome after sirolimus-eluting stent implantation. Coron Artery Dis 2011;22:442–6.

27. Grube E, Silber S, Hauptmann KE, et al. TAXUS I: six- and twelve-month results from a randomized, double-blind trial on a slow-release paclitaxel-eluting stent for de novo coronary lesions. Circulation 2003;107:38–42.

28. Stone GW, Ellis SG, Cannon L, et al. Comparison of a polymer-based paclitaxel-eluting stent with a bare metal stent in patients with complex coronary artery disease: a randomized controlled trial. JAMA 2005;294:1215–23.

29. Stone GW, Ellis SG, Cox DA, et al. A polymer-based, paclitaxel-eluting stent in patients with coronary artery disease. N Engl J Med 2004;350:221–31.

30. Moses JW, Mehran R, Nikolsky E, et al. Outcomes with the paclitaxel-eluting stent in patients with acute coronary syndromes: analysis from the TAXUS-IV trial. J Am Coll Cardiol 2005;45:1165–71.

31. Ellis SG, Stone GW, Cox DA, et al. Long-term safety and efficacy with paclitaxel-eluting stents: 5-year final results of the TAXUS IV clinical trial (TAXUS IV-SR: Treatment of De Novo Coronary Disease Using a Single Paclitaxel-Eluting Stent). JACC Cardiovasc Interv 2009;2:1248–59.

32. Di Lorenzo E, De Luca G, Sauro R, et al. The PASEO (PaclitAxel or Sirolimus-Eluting Stent Versus Bare Metal Stent in Primary Angioplasty) randomized trial. JACC Cardiovasc Interv 2009;2:515–23.

33. Di Lorenzo E, Sauro R, Varricchio A, et al. Long-term outcome of drug-eluting stents compared with bare metal stents in ST-segment elevation myocardial infarction: results of the Paclitaxel- or Sirolimus-Eluting Stent Versus Bare Metal Stent in Primary Angioplasty (PASEO) randomized trial. Circulation 2009;120:964–72.

34. Ong AT, Serruys PW, Aoki J, et al. The unrestricted use of paclitaxel- versus sirolimus-eluting stents for coronary artery disease in an unselected population: one-year results of the Taxus-Stent Evaluated at Rotterdam Cardiology Hospital (T-SEARCH) registry. J Am Coll Cardiol 2005;45:1135–41.

35. Daemen J, Tsuchida K, Stefanini GG, et al. Two-year clinical follow-up of the unrestricted use of the paclitaxel-eluting stent compared to the sirolimus-eluting stent as part of the Taxus-Stent Evaluated at Rotterdam Cardiology Hospital (T-SEARCH) registry. EuroIntervention 2006;2:330–7.

36. Lansky AJ, Costa RA, Mooney M, et al. Gender-based outcomes after paclitaxel-eluting stent implantation in patients with coronary artery disease. J Am Coll Cardiol 2005;45:1180–5.

37. Turco MA, Ormiston JA, Popma JJ, et al. Polymer-based, paclitaxel-eluting TAXUS Liberté stent in de novo lesions: the pivotal TAXUS ATLAS trial. J Am Coll Cardiol 2007;49:1676–83.

38. Turco MA, Ormiston JA, Popma JJ, et al. Reduced risk of restenosis in small vessels and reduced risk of myocardial infarction in long lesions with the new thin-strut TAXUS Liberté stent: 1-year results from the TAXUS ATLAS program. JACC Cardiovasc Interv 2008;1:699–709.

39. Ormiston JA, Turco MA, Hall JJ, et al. Long-term benefit of the TAXUS Liberté stent in small vessels and long lesions. TASIUS ATLAS program. Circ J 2011;75:1120–9.

40. Mikhail GW, Gerber RT, Cox DA, et al. Influence of sex on long-term outcomes after percutaneous coronary intervention with the paclitaxel-eluting coronary stent: results of the "TAXUS Woman" analysis. JACC Cardiovasc Interv 2010;3:1250–9.

41. Abbott JD, Vlachos HA, Selzer F, et al. Gender-based outcomes in percutaneous coronary intervention with drug-eluting stents (from the National Heart, Lung, and Blood Institute Dynamic Registry). Am J Cardiol 2007;99:626–31.

42. Thompson CA, Kaplan AV, Friedman BJ, et al. Gender-based differences of percutaneous coronary intervention in the drug-eluting stent era. Catheter Cardiovasc Interv 2006;67:25–31.

43. Onuma Y, Kukreja N, Daemen J, et al. Impact of sex on 3-year outcome after percutaneous coronary intervention using bare-metal and drug-eluting stents in previously untreated coronary artery disease: insights from the RESEARCH (Rapamycin-Eluting Stent Evaluated at Rotterdam Cardiology Hospital) and T-SEARCH (Taxus-Stent Evaluated at Rotterdam Cardiology Hospital) Registries. JACC Cardiovasc Interv 2009;2:603–10.

44. Kereiakes DJ, Cox DA, Hermiller JB, et al. Usefulness of a cobalt chromium coronary stent alloy. Am J Cardiol 2003;92:463–6.

45. Kastrati A, Mehilli J, Dirschinger J, et al. Intracoronary stenting and angiographic results: strut thickness effect on restenosis outcome (ISAR-STEREO) trial. Circulation 2001;103:2816–21.

46. Khattab AA, Windecker S. Drug-eluting stents: limitations of early generation and progress with newer generation devices. Minerva Med 2010;101:9–23.

47. Fajadet J, Wijns W, Laarman GJ, et al. Randomized, double-blind, multicenter study of the Endeavor zotarolimus-eluting phosphorylcholine-encapsulated stent for treatment of native coronary artery lesions: clinical and angiographic results of the ENDEAVOR II trial. Circulation 2006;114:798–806.

48. Kandzari DE, Leon MB, Popma JJ, et al. Comparison of zotarolimus-eluting and sirolimus-eluting stents in patients with native coronary artery disease: a randomized controlled trial. J Am Coll Cardiol 2006;48:2440–7.

49. Leon MB, Mauri L, Popma JJ, et al. A randomized comparison of the ENDEAVOR zotarolimus-eluting stent versus the TAXUS paclitaxel-eluting stent in de novo native coronary lesions 12-month outcomes from the ENDEAVOR IV trial. J Am Coll Cardiol 2010; 55:543–54.

50. Leon MB, Nikolsky E, Cutlip DE, et al. Improved late clinical safety with zotarolimus-eluting stents compared with paclitaxel-eluting stents in patients with de novo coronary lesions: 3-year follow-up from the ENDEAVOR IV (Randomized Comparison of Zotarolimus- and Paclitaxel-Eluting Stents in Patients With Coronary Artery Disease) trial. JACC Cardiovasc Interv 2010;3:1043–50.

51. Kandzari DE, Mauri L, Popma JJ, et al. Late-term clinical outcomes with zotarolimus- and sirolimus-eluting stents. 5-year follow-up of the ENDEAVOR III (A Randomized Controlled Trial of the Medtronic Endeavor Drug [ABT-578] Eluting Coronary Stent System Versus the Cypher Sirolimus-Eluting Coronary Stent System in De Novo Native Coronary Artery Lesions). JACC Cardiovasc Interv 2011;4: 543–50.

52. Brown RA, Williams M, Barker CM, et al. Sex-specific outcomes following revascularization with zotarolimus-eluting stents: comparison of angiographic and late-term clinical results. Catheter Cardiovasc Interv 2010;76:804–13.

53. Meredith IT, Worthley S, Whitbourn R, et al. Clinical and angiographic results with the next-generation resolute stent system: a prospective, multicenter, first-in-human trial. JACC Cardiovasc Interv 2009;2: 977–85.

54. Udipi K, Melder RJ, Chen M, et al. The next generation Endeavor Resolute Stent: role of the BioLinx Polymer System. EuroIntervention 2007;3: 137–9.

55. Serruys PW, Silber S, Garg S, et al. Comparison of zotarolimus-eluting and everolimus-eluting coronary stents. N Engl J Med 2010;363:136–46.

56. Silber S, Windecker S, Vranckx P, et al. Unrestricted randomised use of two new generation drug-eluting coronary stents: 2-year patient-related versus stent-related outcomes from the RESOLUTE All Comers trial. Lancet 2011;377:1241–7.

57. Yeung AC, Leon MB, Jain A, et al. Clinical evaluation of the Resolute zotarolimus-eluting coronary stent system in the treatment of de novo lesions in native coronary arteries: the RESOLUTE US clinical trial. J Am Coll Cardiol 2011;57:1778–83.

58. Serruys PW, Ong AT, Piek JJ, et al. A randomized comparison of a durable polymer everolimus-eluting stent with a bare metal coronary stent: the SPIRIT first trial. EuroIntervention 2005;1:58–65.

59. Serruys PW, Ruygrok P, Neuzner J, et al. A randomised comparison of an everolimus-eluting coronary stent with a paclitaxel-eluting coronary stent: the SPIRIT II trial. EuroIntervention 2006;2: 286–94.

60. Stone GW, Midei M, Newman W, et al. Comparison of an everolimus-eluting stent and a paclitaxel-eluting stent in patients with coronary artery disease: a randomized trial. JAMA 2008;299:1903–13.

61. Stone GW, Rizvi A, Newman W, et al. Everolimus-eluting versus paclitaxel-eluting stents in coronary artery disease. N Engl J Med 2010;362:1663–74.

62. Garg S, Serruys P, Onuma Y, et al. 3-year clinical follow-up of the XIENCE V everolimus-eluting coronary stent system in the treatment of patients with de novo coronary artery lesions: the SPIRIT II trial (Clinical Evaluation of the Xience V Everolimus Eluting Coronary Stent System in the Treatment of Patients with de novo Native Coronary Artery Lesions). JACC Cardiovasc Interv 2009;2:1190–8.

63. Garg S, Serruys PW, Miquel-Hebert K. Four-year clinical follow-up of the XIENCE V everolimus-eluting coronary stent system in the treatment of patients with de novo coronary artery lesions: the SPIRIT II trial. Catheter Cardiovasc Interv 2011;77: 1012–7.

64. Applegate RJ, Yaqub M, Hermiller JB, et al. Long-term (three-year) safety and efficacy of everolimus-eluting stents compared to paclitaxel-eluting stents (from the SPIRIT III Trial). Am J Cardiol 2011;107: 833–40.

65. Kedhi E, Joesoef KS, McFadden E, et al. Second-generation everolimus-eluting and paclitaxel-eluting stents in real-life practice (COMPARE): a randomised trial. Lancet 2010;375:201–9.

66. Lansky AJ, Ng VG, Mutlu H, et al. Gender-based evaluation of the XIENCE V everolimus-eluting coronary stent system: clinical and angiographic results from the SPIRIT III randomized trial. Catheter Cardiovasc Interv 2009;74:719–27.

67. Ng VG, Lansky AJ, Hermiller JB, et al. Three-year results of safety and efficacy of the everolimus-eluting coronary stent in women (from the SPIRIT III randomized clinical trial). Am J Cardiol 2011; 107:841–8.

68. Seth A, Serruys PW, Lansky A, et al. A pooled gender based analysis comparing the XIENCE V(R) everolimus-eluting stent and the TAXUS paclitaxel-eluting stent in male and female patients with coronary artery disease, results of the SPIRIT II and SPIRIT III studies: two-year analysis. EuroIntervention 2010;5:788–94.

69. Windecker S. SPIRIT Women randomized comparison between everolimus-eluting and sirolimus-eluting stents 9 month angiographic and 1 year clinical follow-up results. Paris: EuroPCR; 2011.

70. Morice MC. The SPIRIT Women clinical trial: one year clinical follow-up. European Society of Cardiology Congress 2010. Stockholm (Sweden), January 9, 2010.

71. Wilson GJ, Nakazawa G, Schwartz RS, et al. Comparison of inflammatory response after implantation of sirolimus- and paclitaxel-eluting stents in porcine coronary arteries. Circulation 2009;120: 141–9, 1–2.

72. Virmani R, Guagliumi G, Farb A, et al. Localized hypersensitivity and late coronary thrombosis secondary to a sirolimus-eluting stent: should we be cautious? Circulation 2004;109:701–5.

73. Nakazawa G, Finn AV, Vorpahl M, et al. Coronary responses and differential mechanisms of late stent thrombosis attributed to first-generation sirolimus- and paclitaxel-eluting stents. J Am Coll Cardiol 2011;57:390–8.

74. O'Brien BJ, Stinson JS, Larsen SR, et al. A platinum-chromium steel for cardiovascular stents. Biomaterials 2010;31:3755–61.

75. Wilson GJ, Huibregtse BA, Stejskal EA, et al. Vascular response to a third generation everolimus-eluting stent. EuroIntervention 2010;6:512–9.

76. Kereiakes DJ, Cannon LA, Feldman RL, et al. Clinical and angiographic outcomes after treatment of de novo coronary stenoses with a novel platinum chromium thin-strut stent: primary results of the PERSEUS (Prospective Evaluation in a Randomized Trial of the Safety and Efficacy of the Use of the TAXUS Element Paclitaxel-Eluting Coronary Stent System) trial. J Am Coll Cardiol 2010;56:264–71.

77. Cannon LA, Kereiakes DJ, Mann T, et al. A prospective evaluation of the safety and efficacy of TAXUS Element paclitaxel-eluting coronary stent implantation for the treatment of de novo coronary artery lesions in small vessels: the PERSEUS Small Vessel trial. EuroIntervention 2011;6:920–7, 1–2.

78. ION monorail over-the-wire paclitaxel-eluting chromium coronary stent system [package insert]. Natick, MA: Boston Scientific Corporation; 2010.

79. Windecker S, Serruys PW, Wandel S, et al. Biolimus-eluting stent with biodegradable polymer versus sirolimus-eluting stent with durable polymer for coronary revascularisation (LEADERS): a randomised non-inferiority trial. Lancet 2008;372:1163–73.

80. Garg S, Sarno G, Serruys PW, et al. The twelve-month outcomes of a biolimus eluting stent with a biodegradable polymer compared with a sirolimus eluting stent with a durable polymer. EuroIntervention 2010;6:233–9.

81. Danzi GB, Maurice M, Mauri F, et al. Nobori Female Study—clinical outcomes at 12 months. J Am Coll Cardiol 2010;55:A194.

82. Ormiston JA, Serruys PW. Bioabsorbable coronary stents. Circ Cardiovasc Interv 2009;2:255–60.

83. Tanimoto S, Serruys PW, Thuesen L, et al. Comparison of in vivo acute stent recoil between the bioabsorbable everolimus-eluting coronary stent and the everolimus-eluting cobalt chromium coronary stent: insights from the ABSORB and SPIRIT trials. Catheter Cardiovasc Interv 2007;70: 515–23.

84. Dudek D, Onuma Y, Ormiston JA, et al. Four-year clinical follow-up of the ABSORB everolimus-eluting bioresorbable vascular scaffold in patients with de novo coronary artery disease: the ABSORB trial. EuroIntervention 2011;7(9):1060–1.

85. Serruys PW, Ormiston JA, Onuma Y, et al. A bioabsorbable everolimus-eluting coronary stent system (ABSORB): 2-year outcomes and results from multiple imaging methods. Lancet 2009;373: 897–910.

86. Ormiston JA, Serruys PW, Regar E, et al. A bioabsorbable everolimus-eluting coronary stent system for patients with single de-novo coronary artery lesions (ABSORB): a prospective open-label trial. Lancet 2008;371:899–907.

87. Serruys PW, Onuma Y, Ormiston JA, et al. Evaluation of the second generation of a bioresorbable everolimus drug-eluting vascular scaffold for treatment of de novo coronary artery stenosis: six-month clinical and imaging outcomes. Circulation 2010;122:2301–12.

88. Gomez-Lara J, Brugaletta S, Diletti R, et al. A comparative assessment by optical coherence tomography of the performance of the first and second generation of the everolimus-eluting bioresorbable vascular scaffolds. Eur Heart J 2011;32: 294–304.

89. Serruys PW, Onuma Y, Dudek D, et al. Evaluation of the second generation of a bioresorbable everolimus-eluting vascular scaffold for the treatment of de novo coronary artery stenosis: 12-month clinical and imaging outcomes. J Am Coll Cardiol 2011;58:1578–88.

90. Dhruva SS, Bero LA, Redberg RF. Gender bias in studies for Food and Drug Administration premarket approval of cardiovascular devices. Circ Cardiovasc Qual Outcomes 2011;4:165–71.

# PCI Outcomes in High-Risk Groups (Diabetes Mellitus, Smoker, Chronic Kidney Disease and the Elderly)

Anouska Moynagh, FRACP[a,b],*,
Marie Claude Morice, MD, FESC[b]

**KEYWORDS**

- Gender • PCI • High-risk • Diabetes • Elderly
- Chronic kidney disease • Smoking

---

**Key Points**

- Ischemic heart disease (IHD) is the leading cause of morbidity and mortality in both genders in developed countries.
- For a variety of reasons, women tend to be underinvestigated and underrepresented in clinical trials and, as a result, treatment of IHD in the female population is based largely on assumption.
- IHD in women is a reality and the incidence increases rapidly after menopause.
- Increased age is a significant risk factor in patients undergoing percutaneous coronary intervention (PCI) for a multitude of reasons; the majority of these patients tend to be female with more complex disease and poorer outcomes.
- Outcomes in both genders with diabetes have improved dramatically in the drug-eluting stent (DES) era.
- The risks of short-term and long-term mortality in men and women with chronic kidney disease (CKD) increase as the gradient of renal dysfunction worsens.
- It is possible that female smokers are more likely to develop IHD than female nonsmokers and male smokers.
- Further clinical trials with adequate female representation need to be performed to study the effects of PCI in these high-risk groups.

---

IHD remains the leading cause of morbidity and mortality in both genders in developed countries.[1] Unfortunately many women underestimate the effect of coronary artery disease on their health and, as a result, the female population tends to be underinvestigated for their symptoms, with less-aggressive treatment approaches when compared with the male cohort, leading to perceived worse outcomes in this group. Despite the postulation that women are protected against

---

Disclosures: The authors have no disclosures.
a Department of Cardiology, King's Mill Hospital, Sutton-In-Ashfield, Nottinghamshire, UK
b Institut Cardiovasculaire Paris Sud, 6, Avenue du Noyer Lambert, Massy 91300, Paris, France
* Corresponding author. Institut Cardiovasculaire Paris Sud, 6, Avenue du Noyer Lambert, Massy 91300, Paris, France.
E-mail address: amoynagh@gmail.com

Intervent Cardiol Clin 1 (2012) 197–205
doi:10.1016/j.iccl.2012.02.004

IHD, in reality, the rate of IHD increases 2 to 3 times after menopause.[2]

Previously, medical research in heart disease has been primarily focused on men. It is now recognized that there are significant differences in coronary artery disease between women and men.[3] In addition, many assumptions about women are from studies where the female population is largely underrepresented and in trials that were not designed to account for any gender differences. The majority of PCI trials have enrolled only 15% to 35% of women.[3] Conflicting results from previous studies, some of which demonstrate possible poorer long-term outcomes in women, may play a role in the decision process, resulting in fewer women referred for PCI.[4–6]

This article discusses PCI in high-risk groups and whether a gender difference exists.

## WHAT IS HIGH-RISK PCI?

The risk of major complications and death during PCI is influenced by many factors. Retrospective studies and databases have been used to identify risk factors for adverse events, including angiographic, patient-related, and clinical factors. These factors can be used to identify high-risk patients, to evaluate and discuss the risk/benefit ratio of proceeding with an intervention, to allow for appropriate measures to be taken to minimize the risk of a major complication, and to predict and treat any complications that might occur.

Several clinical factors can be used to identify high-risk PCI. Such factors include age greater than 65, diabetes, CKD multivessel disease, unstable angina (UA) or recent myocardial infarction (MI), and ST segment elevation MI (STEMI) (**Box 1**).

---

**Box 1**
**Patient and clinical factors associated with high-risk PCI**

Presence of left main stem disease or multivessel disease

PCI of more than one lesion

Impaired ejection fraction (<35%)

Age >65 years

UA and/or recent MI

Diabetes

Smoker

Severe concomitant disease

Renal impairment

---

This review addresses patient-related and clinical factors and how those factors influence outcomes in gender, in particular the evidence in women.

## Age

Age-related physiologic changes augment the risk of adverse outcomes with PCI.[7] From a coronary perspective, elderly patients who require revascularization are more likely to have complex, multivessel disease necessitating more-challenging interventions than for young patients.[8,9] Age is also a significant predictor of coronary medial calcification.[10,11] In a cohort of patients from the Cardiovascular Health Study who were evaluated with electron beam tomography, each additional year increase in age was associated with an 11% increase in risk of a coronary calcium score greater than 900.[10] Interventions on calcified plaques are associated with increased frequency of periprocedural complications, decreased procedural success rates, and incomplete stent expansion and, thus, increased rates of restenosis.[12–14] Tortuous vessels, more commonly observed in older adults, increase the difficulty of coronary device deployment and the risk of complications associated with vascular access.[15]

Additional age-related effects, such as declines in the levels and function of circulating progenitor cells, have led to negative vascular remodeling in response to injury.[16] Furthermore, neointimal reconstitution after stent placement is slower and less complete in older patients than in young.[17]

Hemostatic changes can lead to an increased risk of acute thrombosis[17,18] and, conversely, increased risks of bleeding events.[19]

Age-related alterations in the way drugs are distributed and metabolized in the body also present unique challenges for periprocedural and postprocedural medication choice and dosing[20] and may, in part, explain the increased risk of bleeding when antithrombotic drugs are used in the elderly.

Finally, noncardiac comorbid conditions and declines in cognitive function commonly associated with aging play a substantial part in triggering adverse periprocedural outcomes. The risk of acute and long-term adverse outcomes after PCI increases with worsening baseline renal function[21] and age is a significant predictor of contrast-induced nephropathy after PCI.[22] Frailty, as a clinical syndrome stemming from physical functional decline, decreased nutrition, and reduced cognitive and physical resistance to stressors, is increasingly prevalent with age and occurs in more than 25% of individuals over age 85.[23] Frailty is linked with increased morbidity and mortality[24] and is an independent predictor of adverse outcomes.[23] In the setting of PCI, frailty increases a patient's vulnerability to periprocedural sedation and immobilization and contributes to postprocedural morbidity and mortality.[25]

The contemporary in-hospital mortality rate of PCI is generally low in all age groups but continues to be higher in patients over age 65. Age is strongly associated with a worse short-term prognosis and a greater rate of PCI-related complications.[26–28] Patients less than 65 years of age have an expected in-hospital mortality rate of 0.5% whereas in patients over age 75, this rate ranges from 2.2% to 4.0%. The overall complication rate in elderly patients is 9% compared with 6% for the younger cohort. Bleeding and post-PCI renal failure are more common in elderly patients.[28,29]

An early study of octogenarians undergoing PCI between 1994 and 1997 compared this cohort with patients under 80 years of age who received similar intervention and showed a 2-fold to 4-fold increase in the risk of complications in the older age group, including death (3.8% vs 1.1%), MI (1.9% vs 1.3%), stroke (0.58% vs 0.23%), renal failure (3.2% vs 1.0%), and vascular complications (6.7% vs 3.3%) ($P<.001$ for all comparisons).[15]

For patients undergoing elective PCI, mortality in the older age group varied as much as tenfold, depending on the presence of comorbidities.[15]

Comparatively, long-term survival after successful PCI is good, even in the elderly group. In the era of bare metal stents, restenosis occurred in 15% to 30% of successful PCI cases and was not more frequent in the elderly. Long-term relief of symptoms is achievable in most elderly patients presenting with stable angina although patients over age 75 seem to have higher symptom recurrence than younger patients even after PCI.[30]

The National Cardiovascular Data Registry CathPCI Registry studied patients undergoing PCI in the United States between 2001 and 2006. In-hospital mortality decreased in patients greater than 80 years old but mortality remained 5 times higher in this age group than in younger patients (<80 years) (**Fig. 1**).[31] A similar study in mirrored these findings (**Fig. 2**).[32]

Although these studies emphasize the risks of PCI as a function of age, clinicians and patients need to weigh these acute procedural risks against the potential long-term benefits of intervention. In this regard, trials of coronary revascularization have generally shown that patients at high risk derive greater benefit from revascularization than patients at low risk.[20,33–35] The elderly, who have more cardiovascular risk factors (and, therefore, higher risk of subsequent cardiovascular events),

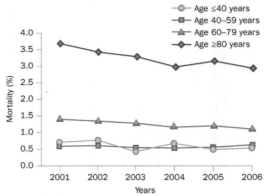

**Fig. 1.** Trends in procedure-related mortality over time in patients undergoing elective PCI (2001–2006). (*From* Bauer T, Mollmann H, Weidinger F, et al. Predictors of hospital mortality in the elderly undergoing percutaneous coronary intervention for acute coronary syndromes and stable angina. Int J Cardiol 2011;151(2):164–9; with permission.)

more severe burden of disease (less ischemic reserve), and less compliant hearts (less tolerant to myocardial oxygen supply-demand mismatch) than younger patients, might derive greater benefit from revascularization.[35–38] Among patients under 75, several randomized clinical trials have helped define the appropriateness of revascularization in specific clinical settings.[39,40]

There are few data available comparing differences between gender groups in the elderly although data show that the majority of elderly patients presenting with coronary artery disease tend to be female and have multivessel coronary artery disease, previous MI, and impaired left ventricular function, which may contribute to poorer outcomes.

### Diabetes Mellitus

Patients with diabetes have a higher incidence for coronary artery disease than the general population.[41] Diabetes is a stronger risk factor for IHD in women than in men with a greater effect on mortality rates.[42–44]

Research has shown that diabetes is associated with rapidly progressive atherosclerosis with smaller vessels, longer lesions, and greater plaque burden. These findings have been associated with worse outcomes after PCI.[45,46] Since the introduction of DESs, randomized trials have shown a marked reduction in the incidence of restenosis compared with previous bare-metal stents[47,48] and some studies have shown good clinical outcomes for DESs in diabetic cohorts.[49,50]

Gender differences have been associated with poorer outcomes since the early days of balloon angioplasty.[51] These differences improved after

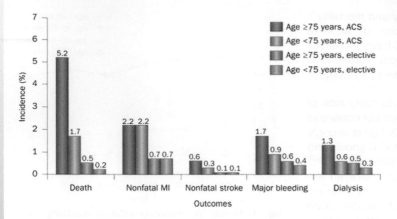

**Fig. 2.** Adverse outcomes after PCI stratified by age and setting. ACS, acute coronary syndromes. (*From* Singh M, Peterson ED, Roe MT, et al. Trends in the association between age and in-hospital mortality after percutaneous coronary intervention: National Cardiovascular Data Registry experience. Circ Cardiovasc Interv 2009;2(1):20–6; with permission.)

the introduction of stents, in particular DESs,[52–55] and gender was no longer independently associated with adverse outcomes, in particular in the low-risk population. A recent study has shown improvements in age-adjusted and cardiovascular mortality rates over the past 30 years with a reduction of 43% in diabetic men, making their outcomes similar to nondiabetic men. There has been no similar reduction visible in women.[56]

There have been observational studies comparing the outcomes in diabetics with respect to gender following PCI in the DES era. Champney and colleagues[42] examined 20,586 PCI procedures during a 13-year period showing substantially improved clinical outcomes in diabetic women after PCI between 1990 and 2003. A Japanese study compared 404 patients (18.3% female) undergoing elective PCI in a single center with follow-up at 4 years. Although women had worse baseline characteristics, the angiographic profiles between the groups were similar with no significant differences in major adverse cardiovascular events (MACE) at 4 years (16.2% vs 15.5%, P = .90) for men and women, respectively (**Fig. 3**).[43]

PCI outcomes of diabetic and nondiabetic men have improved in recent years. Among women, however, diabetics have had greater improvements in outcomes after PCI compared with nondiabetic patients. As a result, diabetes is no longer a stronger risk factor for adverse outcomes after PCI in women than in men.

### Chronic Kidney Disease

CKD alone is an independent risk factor for the development of coronary artery disease and for more severe coronary heart disease (CHD).[57,58] CKD is also associated with an adverse effect on prognosis from cardiovascular disease.[59–61] This includes increased mortality after both acute coronary syndromes and after PCI with or without stenting.[21,62–64] In addition, patients with CKD are more likely to present with atypical symptoms, which may delay diagnosis and adversely affect outcomes.[65]

Patients with CKD are consistently underrepresented in randomized controlled trials of cardiovascular disease.[66] The impact of an invasive strategy has been uncertain in this group. The Swedish Web-System for Enhancement and Development of Evidence-Based Care in Heart Disease Evaluated According to Recommended Therapies (SWEDEHEART) study included a cohort of 23,262 patients hospitalized for non-STEMI (NSTEMI) in Sweden between 2003 and 2006 who were greater than 80 years of age.[67] This contemporary nationwide registry of almost all consecutive patients examined the distribution of CKD and the use of early revascularization after

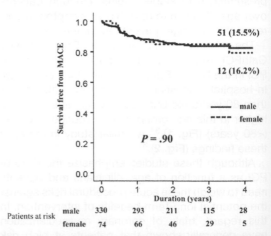

**Fig. 3.** Kaplan-Meier curve for MACE. (*From* Ogita M, Miyauchi K, Dohi T, et al. Gender-based outcomes among patients with diabetes mellitus after percutaneous coronary intervention in the drug-eluting stent era. Int Heart J 2011;52(6):348–52; with permission.)

NSTEMI and evaluated whether early revascularization within 14 days of admission for NSTEMI altered outcomes at all stages of kidney function. Moderate or more advanced CKD was present in 5689 patients (24.4%). After multivariate adjustment, the 1-year mortality in the overall cohort was 36% lower with early revascularization (hazard ratio 0.64; 95% CI, 0.56 to 0.73; $P<.001$). The magnitude of the difference in 1-year mortality was similar in patients with normal estimated glomerular filtration rate and moderate CKD ($P = .001$). The benefit of an invasive therapy was not evident in patients with severe CKD stage IV ($P = .78$) or in those with CKD stage V kidney failure or receiving dialysis ($P = .15$). Early revascularization was associated with 1-year survival in UA/NSTEMI patients with mild to moderate CKD, but no association was observed in those with severe or end-stage kidney disease.

Recently, a collaborative meta-analysis of randomized controlled trials that compared invasive and conservative treatments in UA/NSTEMI was conducted to estimate the effectiveness of early angiography in patients with CKD.[68] This demonstrated that an invasive strategy was associated with a significant reduction in rehospitalization (relative risk [RR] 0.76; 95% CI, 0.66 to 0.87; $P = .001$) at 1 year compared with conservative strategy. The meta-analysis did not show any significant differences with regard to all-cause mortality, nonfatal MI, and the composite of death/nonfatal MI.

The increased risk of mortality associated with mild, moderate, and severe CKD remains evident across studies.[62,68,69] The risks of short-term and long-term mortality are increased as the gradient of renal dysfunction worsens.[68,69]

Additional problems faced in CKD include accelerated atherosclerosis and higher cardiovascular morbidity and mortality.[70,71] Furthermore, CKD is associated with adverse outcome after PCI,[64,72] likely related to endothelial dysfunction, inflammation, and platelet activation. A study by Morel and colleagues, involving 440 patients, included patients with CKD and low responsiveness (LR) to clopidogrel. After 9 months, within the CKD group, the LR status was associated with higher rates of all-cause mortality (25.5% vs 2.8%, $P<.001$), cardiac death (23.5% vs 2.8%, $P<.001$), all-stent thrombosis (19.6% vs 2.7%, $P = .003$), and MACE (33.3% vs 12.3%, $P = .007$). Conversely, in non-CKD patients, the LR status did not affect outcomes. Multivariate analysis identified the interaction between LR and CKD as an independent predictor of cardiac death.

There has been minimal literature on the effect of gender in CKD patients undergoing PCI. One small study examined in-hospital outcomes in 474 chronic dialysis patients undergoing PCI: 36.3% of patients were female. Women had significantly greater rates of in-hospital major adverse cardiac and cerebrovascular events (MACCE) (5.8% vs 1.7%, $P = .013$) and mortality (4.7% vs 0.7%, $P = .006$) than men. After adjustment for the baseline clinical and procedural characteristics, female gender was an independent predictor of MACCE (odds ratio 7.41) and all-cause mortality (odds ratio 13.23).[73]

## Smoking

Worldwide figures reveal that more than 1.1 billion people are smokers, of whom 200 million are women.[74] Every year, smoking-related deaths occur in 1.5 million women.[75] This number is expected to increase to more than 2.5 million female deaths per year and 8 million total deaths per year by 2030 if current smoking patterns persist.[75] A meta-analysis by Huxley and Woodward[76] used prospective cohort studies to determine if women who smoke are at greater risk of CHD than men who smoke. Including data for 3,912,809 individuals, they found that in all age groups, with the exception of the youngest (30–44 years), the effect of smoking on the risk of CHD was greater in women than it was in men, although this difference was only significant for the 60-year-old to 69-year-old age group. Furthermore, when compared with nonsmokers, women who smoke have a 25% greater RR of CHD than male smokers, independent of other cardiovascular risk factors, although the smoking intensity was not taken into account. Knowing that the number of cigarettes smoked per day and the percentage of heavy smokers is generally higher in the male population, the true RR difference between the genders may be underestimated. Mohiuddin and colleagues[77] studied the effects of smoking cessation in patients with cardiovascular disease and found a significant reduction in cardiovascular events at 2 years in the intensive therapy group ($P = .003$) and a similar reduction in mortality ($P = .01$), although a pooled analysis has shown that there was no statistical evidence that the beneficial effects of quitting smoking on subsequent risk of coronary heart disease differed between men and women (RR reduction 0.96, $P = .53$).[76] A further study from Howe and colleagues[78] has shown that women who smoke tend to suffer cardiovascular events at a younger age than female nonsmokers ($P<.001$) and also male smokers. Studying 3588 patients, they found that female smokers were more likely to present with STEMI than their nonsmoking counterparts ($P<.01$), with similar results in the male population. In addition, female smokers had greater risks of cardiovascular events than male smokers both in hospital (11.2% vs 7.7%, $P = .09$) and at 6 months (54.5% vs 33.1%, $P<.001$).

Smoking may have additional harmful effects in women, including blunting of the premenopausal hormonal protection by oxidization of low-density lipoprotein cholesterol.[78] Intravascular ultrasound studies have also shown that culprit lesions in women contain more thrombus.[79] Women typically have smaller coronary arteries and, therefore, may need less thrombus for occlusion, which may potentially magnify the thrombogenic effect of smoking further.

## SUMMARY

Current data suggest that PCI outcomes in women are worse than in men although women are largely underrepresented in clinical trials and, therefore, definitive comparisons are difficult to make. Further clinical trials with higher proportions of female patient recruitment should help to define whether and to what extent a real difference exists further.

## REFERENCES

1. Stramba-Badiale M, Fox KM, Priori SG, et al. Cardiovascular diseases in women: a statement from the policy conference of the European Society of Cardiology. Eur Heart J 2006;27(8):994–1005.

2. Thom T, Haase N, Rosamond W, et al. Heart disease and stroke statistics—2006 update: a report from the American Heart Association Statistics Committee and Stroke Statistics Subcommittee. Circulation 2006;113(6):e85–151.

3. Mikhail GW. Coronary heart disease in women. BMJ 2005;331(7515):467–8.

4. Ellis SG, Roubin GS, King SB 3rd, et al. Angiographic and clinical predictors of acute closure after native vessel coronary angioplasty. Circulation 1988; 77(2):372–9.

5. Watanabe CT, Maynard C, Ritchie JL. Comparison of short-term outcomes following coronary artery stenting in men versus women. Am J Cardiol 2001;88(8):848–52.

6. Argulian E, Patel AD, Abramson JL, et al. Gender differences in short-term cardiovascular outcomes after percutaneous coronary interventions. Am J Cardiol 2006;98(1):48–53.

7. Wang TY, Gutierrez A, Peterson ED. Percutaneous coronary intervention in the elderly. Nat Rev Cardiol 2011;8(2):79–90.

8. Kelsey SF, Miller DP, Holubkov R, et al. Results of percutaneous transluminal coronary angioplasty in patients greater than or equal to 65 years of age (from the 1985 to 1986 National Heart, Lung, and Blood Institute's Coronary Angioplasty Registry). Am J Cardiol 1990;66(15):1033–8.

9. Rizo-Patron C, Hamad N, Paulus R, et al. Percutaneous transluminal coronary angioplasty in octogenarians with unstable coronary syndromes. Am J Cardiol 1990;66(10):857–8.

10. Newman AB, Naydeck BL, Sutton-Tyrrell K, et al. Coronary artery calcification in older adults to age 99: prevalence and risk factors. Circulation 2001; 104(22):2679–84.

11. Sangiorgi G, Rumberger JA, Severson A, et al. Arterial calcification and not lumen stenosis is highly correlated with atherosclerotic plaque burden in humans: a histologic study of 723 coronary artery segments using nondecalcifying methodology. J Am Coll Cardiol 1998;31(1):126–33.

12. Hsu JT, Tamai H, Kyo E, et al. Traditional antegrade approach versus combined antegrade and retrograde approach in the percutaneous treatment of coronary chronic total occlusions. Catheter Cardiovasc Interv 2009;74(4):555–63.

13. Soon KH, Cox N, Wong A, et al. CT coronary angiography predicts the outcome of percutaneous coronary intervention of chronic total occlusion. J Interv Cardiol 2007;20(5):359–66.

14. De Felice F, Fiorilli R, Parma A, et al. Clinical outcome of patients with chronic total occlusion treated with drug-eluting stents. Int J Cardiol 2009; 132(3):337–41.

15. Batchelor WB, Anstrom KJ, Muhlbaier LH, et al. Contemporary outcome trends in the elderly undergoing percutaneous coronary interventions: results in 7,472 octogenarians. National Cardiovascular Network Collaboration. J Am Coll Cardiol 2000;36(3):723–30.

16. Heiss C, Keymel S, Niesler U, et al. Impaired progenitor cell activity in age-related endothelial dysfunction. J Am Coll Cardiol 2005;45(9):1441–8.

17. Becker RC. Thrombotic preparedness in aging: a translatable construct for thrombophilias? J Thromb Thrombolysis 2007;24(3):323–5.

18. Lopes RD, Alexander KP. Antiplatelet therapy in older adults with non-ST-segment elevation acute coronary syndrome: considering risks and benefits. Am J Cardiol 2009;104(Suppl 5):16C–21C.

19. Lakatta EG. Arterial and cardiac aging: major shareholders in cardiovascular disease enterprises: part III: cellular and molecular clues to heart and arterial aging. Circulation 2003;107(3):490–7.

20. Anderson JL, Adams CD, Antman EM, et al. ACC/AHA 2007 guidelines for the management of patients with unstable angina/non-ST-Elevation myocardial infarction: a report of the American College of Cardiology/ American Heart Association Task Force on Practice Guidelines (Writing Committee to Revise the 2002 Guidelines for the Management of Patients With Unstable Angina/Non-ST-Elevation Myocardial Infarction) developed in collaboration with the American College of Emergency Physicians, the Society for Cardiovascular Angiography and Interventions, and

the Society of Thoracic Surgeons endorsed by the American Association of Cardiovascular and Pulmonary Rehabilitation and the Society for Academic Emergency Medicine. J Am Coll Cardiol 2007;50(7):e1–157.

21. Reinecke H, Trey T, Matzkies F, et al. Grade of chronic renal failure, and acute and long-term outcome after percutaneous coronary interventions. Kidney Int 2003;63(2):696–701.

22. Mehran R, Aymong ED, Nikolsky E, et al. A simple risk score for prediction of contrast-induced nephropathy after percutaneous coronary intervention: development and initial validation. J Am Coll Cardiol 2004;44(7):1393–9.

23. Fried LP, Tangen CM, Walston J, et al. Frailty in older adults: evidence for a phenotype. J Gerontol A Biol Sci Med Sci 2001;56(3):M146–56.

24. Buchner DM, Wagner EH. Preventing frail health. Clin Geriatr Med 1992;8(1):1–17.

25. Cohen HJ. In search of the underlying mechanisms of frailty. J Gerontol A Biol Sci Med Sci 2000;55(12): M706–8.

26. Rathore SS, Mehta RH, Wang Y, et al. Effects of age on the quality of care provided to older patients with acute myocardial infarction. Am J Med 2003;114(4): 307–15.

27. Sheifer SE, Rathore SS, Gersh BJ, et al. Time to presentation with acute myocardial infarction in the elderly: associations with race, sex, and socioeconomic characteristics. Circulation 2000;102(14):1651–6.

28. Wennberg DE, Makenka DJ, Sengupta A, et al. Percutaneous transluminal coronary angioplasty in the elderly: epidemiology, clinical risk factors, and in-hospital outcomes. The Northern New England Cardiovascular Disease Study Group. Am Heart J 1999;137(4 Pt 1):639–45.

29. Shaw RE, Anderson HV, Brindis RG, et al. Development of a risk adjustment mortality model using the American College of Cardiology-National Cardiovascular Data Registry (ACC-NCDR) experience: 1998-2000. J Am Coll Cardiol 2002;39(7):1104–12.

30. Hirshfeld JW Jr, Schwartz JS, Jugo R, et al. Restenosis after coronary angioplasty: a multivariate statistical model to relate lesion and procedure variables to restenosis. The M-HEART Investigators. J Am Coll Cardiol 1991;18(3):647–56.

31. Singh M, Peterson ED, Roe MT, et al. Trends in the association between age and in-hospital mortality after percutaneous coronary intervention: National Cardiovascular Data Registry experience. Circ Cardiovasc Interv 2009;2(1):20–6.

32. Bauer T, Mollmann H, Weidinger F, et al. Predictors of hospital mortality in the elderly undergoing percutaneous coronary intervention for acute coronary syndromes and stable angina. Int J Cardiol 2011; 151(2):164–9.

33. Giugliano RP, Lloyd-Jones DM, Camargo CA Jr, et al. Association of unstable angina guideline care with improved survival. Arch Intern Med 2000; 160(12):1775–80.

34. Bhatt DL, Roe MT, Peterson ED, et al. Utilization of early invasive management strategies for high-risk patients with non-ST-segment elevation acute coronary syndromes: results from the CRUSADE Quality Improvement Initiative. JAMA 2004;292(17): 2096–104.

35. Lakatta EG. Changes in cardiovascular function with aging. Eur Heart J 1990;11(Suppl C):22–9.

36. Lakatta E. Aging effects on the vasculature in health: risk factors for cardiovascular disease. Am J Geriatr Cardiol 1994;3(6):11–7.

37. Priebe HJ. The aged cardiovascular risk patient. Br J Anaesth 2000;85(5):763–78.

38. Folkow B, Svanborg A. Physiology of cardiovascular aging. Physiol Rev 1993;73(4):725–64.

39. Coronary artery surgery study (CASS): a randomized trial of coronary artery bypass surgery. Quality of life in patients randomly assigned to treatment groups. Circulation 1983;68(5):951–60.

40. Comparison of coronary bypass surgery with angioplasty in patients with multivessel disease. The Bypass Angioplasty Revascularization Investigation (BARI) Investigators. N Engl J Med 1996;335(4):217–25.

41. Kannel WB, McGee DL. Diabetes and cardiovascular disease. The Framingham study. JAMA 1979; 241(19):2035–8.

42. Champney KP, Veledar E, Klein M, et al. Sex-specific effects of diabetes on adverse outcomes after percutaneous coronary intervention: trends over time. Am Heart J 2007;153(6):970–8.

43. Ogita M, Miyauchi K, Dohi T, et al. Gender-based outcomes among patients with diabetes mellitus after percutaneous coronary intervention in the drug-eluting stent era. Int Heart J 2011;52(6): 348–52.

44. Huxley R, Barzi F, Woodward M. Excess risk of fatal coronary heart disease associated with diabetes in men and women: meta-analysis of 37 prospective cohort studies. BMJ 2006;332(7533):73–8.

45. West NE, Ruygrok PN, Disco CM, et al. Clinical and angiographic predictors of restenosis after stent deployment in diabetic patients. Circulation 2004; 109(7):867–73.

46. Jensen LO, Thayssen P, Mintz GS, et al. Intravascular ultrasound assessment of remodelling and reference segment plaque burden in type-2 diabetic patients. Eur Heart J 2007;28(14):1759–64.

47. Morice MC, Serruys PW, Sousa JE, et al. A randomized comparison of a sirolimus-eluting stent with a standard stent for coronary revascularization. N Engl J Med 2002;346(23):1773–80.

48. Laarman GJ, Suttorp MJ, Dirksen MT, et al. Paclitaxel-eluting versus uncoated stents in primary percutaneous coronary intervention. N Engl J Med 2006;355(11):1105–13.

49. Daemen J, Garcia-Garcia HM, Kukreja N, et al. The long-term value of sirolimus- and paclitaxel-eluting stents over bare metal stents in patients with diabetes mellitus. Eur Heart J 2007;28(1): 26–32.

50. Garg P, Normand SL, Silbaugh TS, et al. Drug-eluting or bare-metal stenting in patients with diabetes mellitus: results from the Massachusetts Data Analysis Center Registry. Circulation 2008; 118(22):2277–85, 7p following 2285.

51. Cowley MJ, Mullin SM, Kelsey SF, et al. Sex differences in early and long-term results of coronary angioplasty in the NHLBI PTCA Registry. Circulation 1985;71(1):90–7.

52. Thompson CA, Kaplan AV, Friedman BJ, et al. Gender-based differences of percutaneous coronary intervention in the drug-eluting stent era. Catheter Cardiovasc Interv 2006;67(1):25–31.

53. Onuma Y, Kukreja N, Daemen J, et al. Impact of sex on 3-year outcome after percutaneous coronary intervention using bare-metal and drug-eluting stents in previously untreated coronary artery disease: insights from the RESEARCH (Rapamycin-Eluting Stent Evaluated at Rotterdam Cardiology Hospital) and T-SEARCH (Taxus-Stent Evaluated at Rotterdam Cardiology Hospital) Registries. JACC Cardiovasc Interv 2009;2(7):603–10.

54. Lansky AJ, Costa RA, Mooney M, et al. Gender-based outcomes after paclitaxel-eluting stent implantation in patients with coronary artery disease. J Am Coll Cardiol 2005;45(8):1180–5.

55. Solinas E, Nikolsky E, Lansky AJ, et al. Gender-specific outcomes after sirolimus-eluting stent implantation. J Am Coll Cardiol 2007;50(22):2111–6.

56. Gregg EW, Gu Q, Cheng YJ, et al. Mortality trends in men and women with diabetes, 1971 to 2000. Ann Intern Med 2007;147(3):149–55.

57. Sarnak MJ, Levey AS, Schoolwerth AC, et al. Kidney disease as a risk factor for development of cardiovascular disease: a statement from the American Heart Association Councils on Kidney in Cardiovascular Disease, High Blood Pressure Research, Clinical Cardiology, and Epidemiology and Prevention. Circulation 2003;108(17):2154–69.

58. Chen J, Muntner P, Hamm LL, et al. The metabolic syndrome and chronic kidney disease in U.S. adults. Ann Intern Med 2004;140(3):167–74.

59. Muntner P, He J, Hamm L, et al. Renal insufficiency and subsequent death resulting from cardiovascular disease in the United States. J Am Soc Nephrol 2002;13(3):745–53.

60. Drey N, Roderick P, Mullee M, et al. A population-based study of the incidence and outcomes of diagnosed chronic kidney disease. Am J Kidney Dis 2003;42(4):677–84.

61. Shlipak MG, Stehman-Breen C, Vittinghoff E, et al. Creatinine levels and cardiovascular events in women with heart disease: do small changes matter? Am J Kidney Dis 2004;43(1):37–44.

62. Shlipak MG, Heidenreich PA, Noguchi H, et al. Association of renal insufficiency with treatment and outcomes after myocardial infarction in elderly patients. Ann Intern Med 2002;137(7):555–62.

63. Al Suwaidi J, Reddan DN, Williams K, et al. Prognostic implications of abnormalities in renal function in patients with acute coronary syndromes. Circulation 2002;106(8):974–80.

64. Best PJ, Lennon R, Ting HH, et al. The impact of renal insufficiency on clinical outcomes in patients undergoing percutaneous coronary interventions. J Am Coll Cardiol 2002;39(7):1113–9.

65. Sosnov J, Lessard D, Goldberg RJ, et al. Differential symptoms of acute myocardial infarction in patients with kidney disease: a community-wide perspective. Am J Kidney Dis 2006;47(3):378–84.

66. Coca SG, Krumholz HM, Garg AX, et al. Underrepresentation of renal disease in randomized controlled trials of cardiovascular disease. JAMA 2006; 296(11):1377–84.

67. Szummer K, Lundman P, Jacobson SH, et al. Influence of renal function on the effects of early revascularization in non-ST-elevation myocardial infarction: data from the Swedish Web-System for Enhancement and Development of Evidence-Based Care in Heart Disease Evaluated According to Recommended Therapies (SWEDEHEART). Circulation 2009;120(10):851–8.

68. Charytan DM, Wallentin L, Lagerqvist B, et al. Early angiography in patients with chronic kidney disease: a collaborative systematic review. Clin J Am Soc Nephrol 2009;4(6):1032–43.

69. Fox CS, Muntner P, Chen AY, et al. Use of evidence-based therapies in short-term outcomes of ST-segment elevation myocardial infarction and non-ST-segment elevation myocardial infarction in patients with chronic kidney disease: a report from the National Cardiovascular Data Acute Coronary Treatment and Intervention Outcomes Network registry. Circulation 2010;121(3): 357–65.

70. Manjunath G, Tighiouart H, Ibrahim H, et al. Level of kidney function as a risk factor for atherosclerotic cardiovascular outcomes in the community. J Am Coll Cardiol 2003;41(1):47–55.

71. Go AS, Chertow GM, Fan D, et al. Chronic kidney disease and the risks of death, cardiovascular events, and hospitalization. N Engl J Med 2004; 351(13):1296–305.

72. Chew DP, Lincoff AM, Gurm H, et al. Bivalirudin versus heparin and glycoprotein IIb/IIIa inhibition among patients with renal impairment undergoing percutaneous coronary intervention (a subanalysis of the REPLACE-2 trial). Am J Cardiol 2005;95(5): 581–5.

73. Parikh PB, Jeremias A, Naidu SS, et al. Effect of gender and race on outcomes in dialysis-dependent

patients undergoing percutaneous coronary intervention. Am J Cardiol 2011;107(9):1319–23.

74. WHO. Tobacco or health: a global status report. Geneva (Switzerland): World Health Organisation; 1997.

75. WHO. WHO report on the global tobacco epidemic, 2008: the MPOWER package. Geneva (Switzerland): World Health Organisation; 2008.

76. Huxley RR, Woodward M. Cigarette smoking as a risk factor for coronary heart disease in women compared with men: a systematic review and meta-analysis of prospective cohort studies. Lancet 2011;378(9799):1297–305.

77. Mohiuddin SM, Mooss AN, Hunter CB, et al. Intensive smoking cessation intervention reduces mortality in high-risk smokers with cardiovascular disease. Chest 2007;131(2):446–52.

78. Howe M, Leidal A, Montgomery D, et al. Role of cigarette smoking and gender in acute coronary syndrome events. Am J Cardiol 2011;108(10):1382–6.

79. Fujii K, Kobayashi Y, Mintz GS, et al. Intravascular ultrasound assessment of ulcerated ruptured plaques: a comparison of culprit and nonculprit lesions of patients with acute coronary syndromes and lesions in patients without acute coronary syndromes. Circulation 2003;108(20):2473–8.

# Vascular Complications in Women and the Radial Approach

Ramya Smitha Suryadevara, MD*,
Kimberly A. Skelding, MD, FSCAI

## KEYWORDS

- Vascular complications • Radial access
- Gender differences • Women • Radial approach
- Percutaneous coronary intervention

Percutaneous coronary intervention (PCI) is an important treatment option for symptomatic coronary artery disease. Bleeding and vascular complications remain high because of the invasive nature and concomitant use of antithrombotic and antiplatelet agents. Bleeding is associated with significant morbidity and mortality. Such complications (**Table 1**) also expose patients to discomfort, longer length of stay in hospital, and excessive consumption of resources.

## GENDER DIFFERENCES

Higher complication rates and mortality are reported in women undergoing PCIs in several studies. A large study by Tavris and colleagues,[1] based on 166,680 patients enrolled in the American College of Cardiology—National Cardiovascular Data Registry (ACC-NCDR) from 1998 to 2001, found that female sex was the strongest predictor of vascular complications (relative risk [RR], 2.18; $P<.001$) and death (RR, 2.59; $P<.001$) compared with their male counterparts. Lansky and colleagues[2] analyzed 14 studies (**Fig. 1**) including a total of 44,264 women and 92,886 men, and showed a vascular complication rate of 5.1% in women compared with 2.6% in men (unadjusted odds ratio [OR], 2.0).

Older age at presentation, higher prevalence of comorbidities, small-caliber arteries, and lower-body surface area have been widely attributed as the causes for higher number of vascular complications in women.[3,4] However, many studies have found that female sex remains an independent risk factor despite adjusting for these variables. In a study of 22,725 consecutive patients enrolled in Blue Cross Blue Shield of Michigan Cardiovascular Consortium, a large multicenter regional consortium, even after adjusting for baseline demographics, comorbidities, clinical presentation, and lesion characteristics, women had a 3-fold increased risk of vascular complications, 2-fold increased risk of contrast-induced nephropathy, and more than twice as many transfusions as men (8.84% vs 3.87%, $P<.0001$).[5]

Several improvements in equipment, technique, and pharmacotherapies have lowered complication rates. The use of vascular closure devices,[1,6–9] small vascular sheaths, improved access techniques such as use of fluoroscopic guidance for femoral access, increased use of radial access, and antithrombotic therapies such as bivalirudin[10] have reduced the complication rate in both men and women. Female sex, however, continues to be a risk factor for vascular complications, and the use of these methods does not level the playing field. A study of 13,653 female and 32,334 male consecutive cases, from 2002 to 2007, in the Northern New England PCI Registry showed that although there was more than 50% reduction in

Department of Cardiology, Geisinger Medical Center, 100 Academy Avenue, Danville, PA 17821, USA
* Corresponding author.
E-mail address: rssuryadevara@geisinger.edu

Intervent Cardiol Clin 1 (2012) 207–211
doi:10.1016/j.iccl.2012.01.004

interventional.theclinics.com

## Table 1
### Incidence of major vascular complications after PCI

| Complication | Incidence (%) |
| --- | --- |
| Bleeding including entry site bleeding, local hematoma, and retroperitoneal hemorrhage | 3.44 |
| Dissection | 0.18 |
| Pseudoaneurysm | 0.32 |
| Arteriovenous fistula formation | 0.02 |
| Occlusion by thrombus formation | 0.12 |
| Entry-site infection | 0.03 |
| Surgical vascular device removal | 0.08 |

*Data from* Tavris DR, Gallauresi BA, Lin BJ, et al. Risk of local adverse events following cardiac catheterization by hemostasis device use and gender. J Invasive Cardiol 2004;16:459–64.

complication rates in both men and women, female sex remained a significant predictor for increased risk until the end of the study period (OR, 2.6; 95% confidence interval [CI], 1.74–3.91).[11]

## CLINICAL AND PROCEDURAL PREDICTORS

In a study of 13,653 patients enrolled in the Northern New England PCI Registry, older age, renal failure, presentation with non–ST-segment myocardial infarction or cardiogenic shock, and

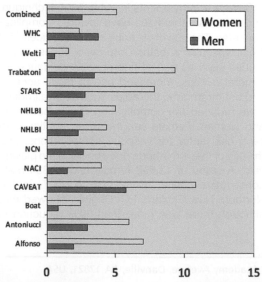

**Fig. 1.** Meta-analysis of vascular complications in patients undergoing PCI: women versus men. (*Data from* Refs.[2,4,23–33])

use of larger sheaths independently predicted a higher incidence of vascular complications in women.[11] In the same study the investigators noted a decreased risk of vascular complications in women with dyslipidemia, use of vascular closure devices, women with prior history of revascularization, and use of bivalirudin.[11] Another study of 4157 women enrolled in the Acute Catheterization and Urgent Intervention Triage strategy (ACUITY) trial, age older than 75 years, anemia, creatinine clearance less than 60 mL/min, elevated cardiac biomarkers, electrocardiographic changes at presentation, diabetes mellitus, and treatment with heparin and GP IIb/IIIa versus bivalirudin alone were shown to be predictors of 30-day major bleeding after PCI.[12]

## USE OF ANTITHROMBOTIC AGENTS IN WOMEN

In a pooled analysis of the Evaluation of 7E3 for the Prevention of Ischemic Complications (EPIC), Evaluation in Percutaneous Transluminal Coronary Angioplasty to Improve Long-Term Outcome with Abciximab GP IIb/IIIa Blockade (EPILOG), and Evaluation of Platelet IIb/IIIa Inhibitor for Stenting (EPISTENT) trials, abciximab reduced the 30-day rate of major adverse cardiovascular events in women from 12.5% to 6.5% (P<.0001). However, similar rates of major bleeding were noted in women with and without abciximab (3% vs 2.9%; P = .96). In addition, there was a significant increase in the risk of minor bleeding with abciximab versus placebo (6.7% vs 4.7%; P = .01).[13]

Several studies noted that the use of glycoprotein IIb/IIIa inhibitors during PCI is not an independent risk factor for major vascular complications in women.[13–15] However, the use of bivalirudin instead of unfractionated heparin during elective PCI did reduce the risk of bleeding in both women and men, although women continued to have a higher rate of bleeding overall.[16]

## RADIAL APPROACH

Since Campeau and Kiemeneij published their successful series on diagnostic coronary angiography and PCI using radial access, the cumulative favorable evidence over the past 2 decades has demonstrated that the radial artery is the preferred site of vascular access to reduce bleeding risk and decrease both morbidity and mortality. The Radial Versus Femoral Access for Coronary Intervention (RIVAL) trial, a large randomized, parallel group multicenter trial, found the radial-artery approach to be as effective as the femoral approach, but with fewer vascular complications.[17] In a large

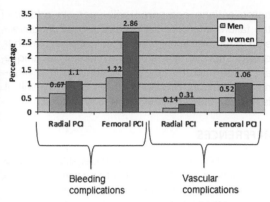

Bleeding complications    Vascular complications

**Fig. 2.** Bleeding and vascular complications following radial PCI versus femoral PCI in men and women. (*Data from* Pristipino C, Pelliccia F, Granatelli A, et al. Comparison of access-related bleeding complications in women versus men undergoing percutaneous coronary catheterization using the radial vs femoral artery. Am J Cardiol 2007;99:1216–21.)

meta-analysis of 12 studies (n = 3244), the incidence of vascular complications after transradial procedures was significantly lower than that seen in transfemoral cases (0.3% vs 2.8%, P<.001).[18] As yet there has not been a randomized trial demonstrating superiority of the femoral access.

In fact, Pristipino and colleagues[19] prospectively followed 3261 consecutive percutaneous coronary procedures and noted that in women, no major bleeding occurred after 299 radial access procedures compared with 25 major bleeding episodes after 601 femoral access procedures (P = .0008). Incidence of minor hemorrhages was also noted to be less in women who underwent radial access in comparison with femoral access (6.4%, vs 39.4%, respectively, P = .00001).[19] However, women who underwent radial access procedures

still had a higher incidence of bleeding complications compared with men who underwent radial access procedures (OR, 4.5; 95% CI, 2.2–9.0).[19] Although women continued having more numerous vascular/bleeding complications in the trial, the radial approach, when compared with the femoral approach, provided greater benefit to women than to men (**Fig. 2**).[19]

A study of 1348 patients with acute coronary syndrome enrolled in the EArly discharge after Stenting of coronarY arteries (EASY) trial, undergoing transradial PCI with all subjects pretreated with aspirin and clopidogrel (Plavix) and receiving 70 units per kilogram of heparin and abciximab, there was similar procedural duration. Regardless of complexity and despite the use of smaller sheath size in women, more hematomas were noted (**Table 2**). Female sex was the only independent predictor for mild or moderate hematoma (OR, 4.4; 95% CI, 2.49–7.81; P<.0001).[20]

One potential issue is that women are more likely than men to require crossover to a second access site after the radial access (14% vs 1.7%). However, operators who used the transradial approach as primary access completed the procedure successfully in more than 90% of patients.[19] Other studies found similar results, including a study of a total of 2100 patients who underwent transradial PCI.[21] The investigators noted that female sex is a univariate predictor (**Table 3**) of transradial PCI failure (OR, 1.84; 95% CI, 1.15–2.92; P = .01); however, women comprised only 17% of the enrollment. The major mechanisms and causes of transradial PCI failure noted in this study are inadequate arterial puncture (13%), arterial spasm (33%), arterial dissection (10%), artery loop/tortuosity (6%), artery stenosis (1%), and subclavian tortuosity (18%). Once

**Table 2**
**Thirty-day events after radial PCI in the EASY trial: men versus women**

|  | Women (n = 298; 22%) | Men (n = 1050; 78%) | P Value |
|---|---|---|---|
| Death | 0 (0%) | 2 (0.2%) | 1.00 |
| MI | 9 (3.0%) | 37 (3.5%) | .86 |
| Urgent revascularization (CABG and PCI) | 1 (0.3%) | 13 (1.2%) | .33 |
| Major bleeding | 7 (2.4%) | 12 (1.1%) | .16 |
| Thrombocytopenia (<100,000/μL) | 2 (0.7%) | 17 (1.6%) | .28 |
| Any transfusion | 5 (1.7%) | 10 (1.0%) | .34 |
| Repeat hospitalization | 17 (5.7%) | 47 (4.5%) | .36 |
| Hematoma | 67 (22%) | 81 (5.8%) | <.0001 |

*Abbreviations:* CABG, coronary artery bypass grafting; MI, myocardial infarction.
*Data from* Tizón-Marcos H, Bertrand OF, Rodés-Cabau J, et al. Impact of female gender and transradial coronary stenting with maximal antiplatelet therapy on bleeding and ischemic outcomes. Am Heart J 2009;157:740–5.

**Table 3**
**Predictors (univariate) of transradial PCI failure**

| Predictors | Odds Ratio | P Value |
|---|---|---|
| Age ≥75 years | 4.41 (95% CI 2.732–7.12) | <.0001 |
| Female sex | 1.84 (95% CI 1.15–2.92) | .01 |
| Prior CABG | 4.65 (95% CI 2.34–9.21) | <.0001 |
| Height | 0.96 (95% CI 0.94–0.98) | .001 |

*Abbreviation:* CI, confidence interval.
*Data from* Dehghani P, Mohammed A, Bajaj R, et al. Mechanism and predictors of failed transradial approach for percutaneous coronary interventions. J Am Coll Cardiol 2009;2:1057–64.

access was achieved, 36% of patients had failure of transradial PCI caused by inadequate coronary cannulation requiring a switch to femoral access.[21]

Several strategies have been suggested to overcome the challenges with radial access, including use of nitroglycerin, calcium-channel blockers, proper sedation, and smaller-sized catheters to minimize spasm, as well as proper positioning of patients. Performing radiobrachial angiography in the event of resistance to advancing wire, use of hydrophilic wires to straighten and traverse radial loops, and having the patient take a deep breath to straighten the subclavian and innominate artery and subclavian/innominate aortic junction has also been used to increase success rates. The use of Judkin curves (JR5 and JL3.5) and other specialized curves, such as Tiger, Jacky, and Amplatz, for engaging the coronary arteries is also recommended to achieve an increase in success rates.[22]

In summary, radial access in women reduces complications, and is associated with lower morbidity and mortality rates. Feasibility is improved by simple technical measures, and the technique should be used routinely to lower complication rates. However, there is a learning curve that needs to be overcome to increase the success rate of radial access procedures. The RIVAL study showed that operators who use radial access routinely have the opportunity not only to decrease the bleeding rates but also to potentially decrease mortality.

## SUMMARY

Despite technical advances, vascular complications after PCI, including bleeding, remain higher in women. Compared with femoral access, radial artery access for PCI was shown to have far fewer bleeding complications and a similar success rate. However, even women undergoing transradial access for PCI have higher vascular/bleeding complications compared with men. In addition, the failure rate of radial access, requiring conversion to femoral access, is higher in women. Further quality improvement studies evaluating technique and pharmacotherapy are needed in this high-risk population. Studies such as Safe PCI will, it is hoped, answer some of these questions.

## REFERENCES

1. Tavris DR, Gallauresi BA, Lin BJ, et al. Risk of local adverse events following cardiac catheterization by hemostasis device use and gender. J Invasive Cardiol 2004;16:459–64.
2. Lansky AJ, Hochman JS, Ward PA. Percutaneous coronary intervention and adjunctive pharmacotherapy in women: a statement for healthcare professionals from the American Heart Association. Circulation 2005;111:940–53.
3. Ashby DT, Mehran R, Aymong EA, et al. Comparison of outcomes in men versus women having percutaneous coronary interventions in small coronary arteries. Am J Cardiol 2003;91:979–81, A974, A977.
4. Peterson ED, Lansky AJ, Kramer J, et al. Effect of gender on the outcomes of contemporary percutaneous coronary intervention. Am J Cardiol 2001;88:359–64.
5. Duvernoy CS, Smith DE, Manohar P, et al. Gender differences in adverse outcomes after contemporary percutaneous coronary intervention: an analysis from the Blue Cross Blue Shield of Michigan Cardiovascular Consortium (BMC2) Percutaneous Coronary Intervention Registry. Am Heart J 2010;159(4):677–83.
6. Dauerman HL, Applegate RJ, Cohen DJ. Vascular closure devices: the second decade. J Am Coll Cardiol 2007;50:1617–26.
7. Nikolsky E, Mehran R, Halkin A, et al. Vascular complications associated with arteriotomy closure devices in patients undergoing percutaneous coronary procedures: a meta-analysis. J Am Coll Cardiol 2004;44:1200–9.
8. Applegate RJ, Sacrinty MT, Kutcher MA, et al. Trends in vascular complications after diagnostic cardiac catheterization and percutaneous coronary intervention via the femoral artery, 1998 to 2007. J Am Coll Cardiol 2008;1:317–26.
9. Turi Z. An evidence-based approach to femoral arterial access and closure. Rev Cardiovasc Med 2009;9:7–18.
10. Stone GW, McLaurin BT, Cox DA, et al. ACUITY Investigators. Bivalirudin for patients with acute coronary syndromes. N Engl J Med 2006;355:2203–16.
11. Ahmed B, Piper WD, Malenka D, et al. Significantly improved vascular complications among women undergoing percutaneous coronary intervention: a

report from the Northern New England Percutaneous Coronary Intervention Registry. Circ Cardiovasc Interv 2009;2:423–9.

12. Lansky AJ, Mehran R, Cristea E, et al. Impact of gender and antithrombin strategy on early and late clinical outcomes in patients with non-ST-elevation acute coronary syndromes (from the ACUITY trial). Am J Cardiol 2009;103:1196–203.

13. Cho L, Topol EJ, Balog C, et al. Clinical benefit of glycoprotein IIb/IIIa blockade with abciximab is independent of gender: pooled analysis from EPIC, EPILOG and EPISTENT trials. Evaluation of 7E3 for the Prevention of Ischemic Complications. Evaluation in Percutaneous Transluminal Coronary Angioplasty to Improve Long-Term Outcome with Abciximab GP IIb/IIIa blockade. Evaluation of Platelet IIb/IIIa Inhibitor for Stent. J Am Coll Cardiol 2000;36:381–6.

14. Fernandes LS, Tcheng JE, O'Shea JC, et al. Is glycoprotein IIb/IIIa antagonism as effective in women as in men following percutaneous coronary intervention? Lessons from the ESPRIT study. J Am Coll Cardiol 2002;40:1085–91.

15. Lansky AJ, Pietras C, Costa RA, et al. Gender differences in outcomes after primary angioplasty versus primary stenting with and without abciximab for acute myocardial infarction: results of the Controlled Abciximab and Device Investigation to Lower Late Angioplasty Complications (CADILLAC) trial. Circulation 2005;111:1611–8.

16. Chacko M, Lincoff AM, Wolski KE, et al. Ischemic and bleeding outcomes in women treated with bivalirudin during percutaneous coronary intervention: a subgroup analysis of the Randomized Evaluation in PCI Linking Angiomax to Reduced Clinical Events (REPLACE)-2 trial. Am Heart J 2006;151:1032.e1–7.

17. Jolly SS, Niemela K, Xavier D, et al. Design and rationale of the radial versus femoral access for coronary intervention (RIVAL) trial: a randomized comparison of radial versus femoral access for coronary angiography or intervention in patients with acute coronary syndrome. Am Heart J 2011; 161(2):254–60. E1–4.

18. Agostoni P, Biondi-Zoccai GG, de Benedictis ML, et al. Radial versus femoral approach for percutaneous coronary diagnostic and interventional procedures; systematic overview and meta-analysis of randomized trials [review]. J Am Coll Cardiol 2004; 44:349–56.

19. Pristipino C, Pelliccia F, Granatelli A, et al. Comparison of access-related bleeding complications in women versus men undergoing percutaneous coronary catheterization using the radial versus femoral artery. Am J Cardiol 2007;99:1216–21.

20. Tizón-Marcos H, Bertrand OF, Rodés-Cabau J, et al. Impact of female gender and transradial coronary stenting with maximal antiplatelet therapy on bleeding and ischemic outcomes. Am Heart J 2009;157:740–5.

21. Dehghani P, Mohammed A, Bajaj R, et al. Mechanism and predictors of failed transradial approach for percutaneous coronary interventions. J Am Coll Cardiol 2009;2:1057–64.

22. Rao SV, Cohen MG, Kandzari DE, et al. The transradial approach to percutaneous coronary intervention, historical perspective, current concepts and future directions. J Am Coll Cardiol 2010;55:2187–95.

23. Alfonso F, Hernandez R, Banuelos C, et al. Initial results and long-term clinical and angiographic outcome of coronary stenting in women. Am J Cardiol 2000;86:1380–3 A1385.

24. Antoniucci D, Valenti R, Moschi G, et al. Sex-based differences in clinical and angiographic outcomes after primary angioplasty or stenting for acute myocardial infarction. Am J Cardiol 2001;87:289–93.

25. Baim DS, Cutlip DE, Sharma SK, et al. Final results of the Balloon vs Optimal Atherectomy Trial (BOAT). Circulation 1998;97:322–31.

26. Omoigui NA, Califf RM, Pieper K, et al. Peripheral vascular complications in the Coronary Angioplasty Versus Excisional Atherectomy Trial (CAVEAT-I). J Am Coll Cardiol 1995;26:922–30.

27. Robertson T, Kennard ED, Mehta S, et al. Influence of gender on in-hospital clinical and angiographic outcomes and on one-year follow-up in the New Approaches to Coronary Intervention (NACI) registry. Am J Cardiol 1997;80:26K–39K.

28. Kelsey SF, James M, Holubkov AL, et al. Results of percutaneous transluminal coronary angioplasty in women. 1985-1986 National Heart, Lung, and Blood Institute's Coronary Angioplasty Registry. Circulation 1993;87:720–7.

29. Jacobs AK, Johnston JM, Haviland A, et al. Improved outcomes for women undergoing contemporary percutaneous coronary intervention: a report from the National Heart, Lung, and Blood Institute Dynamic registry. J Am Coll Cardiol 2002;39:1608–14.

30. Leon MB, Baim DS, Popma JJ, et al. A clinical trial comparing three antithrombotic-drug regimens after coronary-artery stenting. Stent Anticoagulation Restenosis Study Investigators. N Engl J Med 1998; 339:1665–71.

31. Bell MR, Garratt KN, Bresnahan JF, et al. Immediate and long-term outcome after directional coronary atherectomy: analysis of gender differences. Mayo Clin Proc 1994;69:723–9.

32. Lansky AJ, Mehran R, Dangas G, et al. New-device angioplasty in women: clinical outcome and predictors in a 7,372-patient registry. Epidemiology 2002; 13:S46–51.

33. Welty FK, Lewis SM, Kowalker W, et al. Reasons for higher in-hospital mortality >24 hours after percutaneous transluminal coronary angioplasty in women compared with men. Am J Cardiol 2001;88:473–7.

# Is Stenting an Appropriate Therapy in Women Presenting with Acute Coronary Syndrome? A Pathologist's Perspective

Masataka Nakano, MD, Fumiyuki Otsuka, MD, PhD,
Renu Virmani, MD*

KEYWORDS

- Stenting • Women • Acute coronary syndrome
- Drug-eluting stents

The definition of acute coronary syndrome (ACS) is based on symptomatic manifestation of patients presenting with myocardial ischemia (ie, reduced blood flow to the heart). The main categories include unstable angina, non-ST elevation myocardial infarction (MI), and ST elevation MI, defined by electrocardiographic changes and by cardiac markers, troponin T and I. According to the American Heart Association and the American College of Cardiology, 5 factors should be considered when assessing the likelihood of myocardial ischemia. These factors include nature of symptoms, history of ischemic heart disease, sex, increasing age, and the number of traditional cardiovascular risk factors present. High-risk factors include worsening angina, prolonged chest pain (>20 minutes), pulmonary edema, hypotension, and arrhythmias. The major cause of myocardial ischemia is coronary atherosclerosis with superimposed luminal thrombosis. Autopsy studies of sudden death victims have elucidated

the main histopathologic nidus of ACS (ie, thrombosis caused by rupture of the fibrous cap and exposure of highly thrombogenic necrotic core to blood flow or by erosion where there is loss of luminal endothelium). Further, as the morphologies of culprit plaque have been extensively studied, there is emerging evidence indicating that there are differences in ACS substrates between genders.

It has been more than 3 decades since the introduction of percutaneous transluminal coronary angioplasty for the treatment of coronary artery disease, and in the last decade there has been revolutionary progress, especially with the introduction of bare metal stents (BMS) and drug-eluting stents (DES), which have significantly improved clinical outcomes by decreasing rates of acute vessel closure and restenosis. Because our facility holds the largest autopsy registry of stents implanted in human coronary arteries, we have reported pathologic changes

Disclosures: Dr Virmani receives consulting fee from Abbott Vascular; Arsenal Medical; Atrium Medical Corporation; Biosensors International; GlaxoSmithKline; Lutonix, Inc.; Medtronic AVE; Abbott Vascular; W.L. Gore. Dr Nakano and Dr Otsuka have no conflict of interest in relation to the topic of this manuscript.
CVPath Institute, 19 Firstfield Road, Gaithersburg, MD 20878, USA
* Corresponding author.
E-mail address: rvirmani@cvpath.org

Intervent Cardiol Clin 1 (2012) 213–221
doi:10.1016/j.iccl.2012.01.003
2211-7458/12/$ – see front matter Published by Elsevier Inc.

observed after stenting, which are attributed to restenosis and thrombosis. Although these data have widened our understanding of the advantages and disadvantages of current devices, little is known about the difference between women and men presenting with ACS. This article reviews pathologic findings from male and female patients who had received coronary stents for ACS and died suddenly with or without complications of stent implantation, at early (<30 days) and late (>30 days) time points after DES implantation.

# HISTOPATHOLOGY OF ACS AND THROMBOSIS
## Plaque Rupture and Erosion of Coronary Artery

The most common substrate underlying the onset of ACS is considered to be the rupture of a vulnerable plaque, which contains a necrotic core and is covered by a fibrous cap (**Fig. 1**). The term thin cap fibroatheroma (TCFA) is used to describe vulnerable plaque, because histomorphometric analysis revealed fibrous cap thickness to be less than 65 μm in 95% of the lesions.[1] Once the disruption of

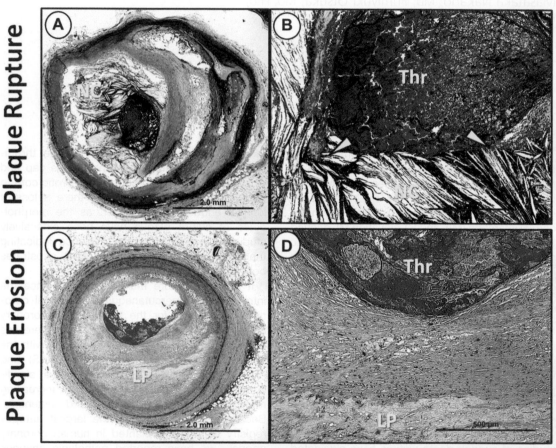

**Fig. 1.** Representative cases of patients dying of plaque rupture and erosion in coronary arteries. (*A, B*) 83-year-old man with history of diabetes and dyslipidemia. The patient presented to the emergency department complaining of shortness of breath and with findings consistent with ST elevation MI; the patient was taken to the catheterization laboratory, where he became unresponsive during femoral line placement and could not be resuscitated. On histologic assessment, there was focal severe coronary atherosclerosis and acute plaque rupture of the proximal right coronary artery (*A*). High-power imaging (*B*) confirmed disruption of the fibrous cap (*arrows*) overlying the necrotic core (NC) with thrombotic occlusion (Thr). (*C, D*) 37-year-old woman with history of hypertension, diabetes, and obesity, and recent complaint of chest pain for 1 week's duration; the patient had a witnessed arrest and could not be resuscitated. At autopsy, focal severe coronary atherosclerosis, plaque erosion with 75% luminal narrowing, and nonocclusive thrombus were identified in the proximal left anterior descending artery (*C*). The vessel size was relatively small. In high-power imaging (*D*), there was neither disruption of fibrous cap nor connection between luminal thrombus and lipid pool (LP) within the plaque.

the fibrous cap occurs in TCFA, the exposure of thrombogenic necrotic materials to blood flow results in a luminal thrombus with or without embolization into distal intramural arteries. The embolus is most often composed of thrombotic fragments and rarely of atherosclerotic debris, both resulting in loss of surrounding myocardium.

Plaque erosion accounts for 30% to 35% of the cases of acute coronary thrombosis identified at autopsy and is regarded as an important substrate in patients presenting with ACS,[2,3] especially young women (see **Fig. 1**). There are clear morphologic differences between rupture and erosion, with plaque erosion having more frequently lesions rich in proteoglycan-versican, hyaluronan, and type III collagen, unlike rupture.[4] In plaque erosion, the thrombus is confined to the luminal surface and in 50% of cases it has an underlying necrotic core. Moreover, erosions generally show smaller internal elastic lamina (IEL) areas compared with ruptures Although IEL area progressively decreased with greater maturation of the thrombus, this relationship is not so stringent when plaques with significant stenosis are examined. These data are in concordance with an earlier study from our laboratory in which marked expansion of the IEL was noted for plaque rupture, whereas erosions showed negative remodeling.[5] Coronary lesions with ruptures from patients dying suddenly are generally more severely narrowed; on the contrary, erosion lesions have less severe luminal narrowing, and are thus less likely to be flow limiting. Also the medial wall is not attenuated, and the IEL and the external elastic lamina are well discerned in erosions, whereas in ruptures the IEL is often lost and the media is attenuated or completely lost.[6]

Coronary thrombi at autopsy show diverse phases of healing dependent on the cause of the underlying culprit plaque. In ruptures, nearly half of thrombi showed a lack of healing characterized by platelets/fibrin with entrapped polymorphonuclear leukocytes without evidence of lysis, whereas the remaining (50%) showed various phases of healing. In contrast, more than 85% of thrombi in erosions showed late stages of healing characterized by inflammatory cell lysis, invasion by smooth muscle cells (SMC) or endothelial cells, or organized layers of SMC and proteoglycans with varying degrees of platelet/fibrin layering.[7] Approximately two-thirds of coronary thrombi in sudden coronary deaths are organizing, particularly in young individuals, especially women, who might require a different strategy of treatment of ACS. In patients presenting with ST elevation MI, thrombus aspirates that were older than 1 day had a poorer prognosis compared with those with fresh thrombus.[8]

## Gender Difference in ACS

Differences between genders is well established in ACS because the incidence of sudden death and acute MI (AMI) is 3 to 4 times less in women than in men,[9] especially in individuals younger than 50 years. Pathologic evidence supporting the important role of gender as reported by Arbustini and colleagues[10] in which erosions accounted for 25% of 291 inhospital-based deaths from AMI, with most erosion occurring in women. We also have shown distinct differences in the incidence of plaque rupture and erosion in women and men in a study of patients dying suddenly from coronary diseases in whom plaque erosion was identified more frequently in women with acute thrombosis (65%) than in men (27%). When the data were stratified by age greater or less than 50 years, there was an 80% incidence of plaque erosion in women less than 50 years of age.[2] Also, in women older than 50 years there was a higher incidence of plaque rupture compared with erosion (**Table 1**). Moreover, Burke and colleagues[11] reported that women dying suddenly with plaque erosion were more often smokers and that dyslipidemia was a predictor of plaque rupture and not erosion. Therefore menopausal status of women has a substantial impact on plaque instability and plaque morphology, thus implying that estrogen may be protective in preventing plaque rupture.[12,13] The molecular and cellular basis

**Table 1**
**Distribution of culprit plaques by gender and age in sudden coronary death cases**

|  | Acute Thrombi | | |
|---|---|---|---|
|  | **Rupture** | **Erosion** | **Calcified Nodule** |
| Men | 64 (68) | 25 (27) | 5 (5) |
| <50 y | 45 (70) | 17 (27) | 2 (3) |
| >50 y | 19 (63) | 8 (27) | 3 (10) |
| Women | 10 (32) | 20 (65) | 1 (3) |
| <50 y | 1 (7) | 14 (93) | 0 (0) |
| >50 y | 9 (56) | 6 (38) | 1 (6) |

Values correspond to the number of cases; those in parentheses are percentages.
*Data from* Virmani R, Kolodgie FD, Burke AP, et al. Lessons from sudden coronary death: a comprehensive morphologic classification scheme for atherosclerotic lesions. Arteriocler Thromb Vasc Biol 2000;20(5):1263–75.

underlying these differences remains mostly un-known; however, it is suggested that estrogen has potential beneficial effects on lipid metabolism, nitric oxide-mediated vasodilatation, and vascular response to the injury.[14] We suspect that vasospasm may be the underlying mechanism of plaque erosion; however, this needs further proof.

## HISTOPATHOLOGY OF STENTED CORONARY ARTERY
### Vessel Healing After Stent Implantation

Vessel healing after stent implantation is analogous to the pattern of wound healing from injury.[15,16] Vascular healing after balloon angioplasty and stenting can be divided into 4 phases with immediate changes consisting of platelets and fibrin deposition with focal acute inflammatory cell infiltrates; these responses are concentrated around stent struts and are observed up to the first month. Within 14 days, granulation tissue is observed, which consists of smooth muscle and endothelial cell proliferation and chronic inflammation. Extracellular proteoglycans matrix is laid down within 1 month and peaks at 6 months. The healing process is complete when complete endothelialization is seen at 3 to 4 months. In BMS, it has been shown that peak neointimal thickening occurs between 6 and 18 months and thereafter there is a decrease as type III collagen is replaced by type I collagen, which cross-links and shrinks along with loss of SMC, resulting in negative remodeling with enlargement of the lumen. However, vessel healing in DES is fundamentally delayed. Fibrin deposition is usually greater in DES compared with BMS in the persistent locations and lasts for a long time. Poor endothelial cell coverage of the lumen is a consistent finding in DES cases even beyond 6 months and may be seen as late as 2 to 3 years after implantation, whereas SMC growth is significantly less.

### Pathology of Restenosis

The early studies of in-stent restenosis after BMS implantation show excessive SMC-rich neointima along with proteoglycan and collagen matrix deposition with capillaries, macrophages, and lymphocytes mostly concentrated around the stent struts.[17] Macrophages secrete cytokines and growth factors that have been shown to induce SMC proliferation and migration in in vitro models.[18,19]

In a larger autopsy cohort study, our group showed that medial destruction and lipid core penetration result in increased inflammation, which is associated with neointimal overgrowth (**Fig. 2**).[20]

This finding suggests that overexpansion of the stent potentially leads to restenosis, involving excessive platelet aggregation, polymorphonuclear leukocyte and macrophage infiltration, granulation tissue, SMC migration and proliferation, and extracellular matrix deposition. Therefore, strategies that reduce medial damage and optimize appropriate stent sizing may lower the frequency of in-stent restenosis.

### Pathology of Stent Thrombosis

The cause of early (<1 month) stent thrombosis includes clinical procedural factors such as stent malapposition, dissection, prolapse of the necrotic core, vessel perforations, and premature cessation of dual antiplatelet therapy; the incidence of early stent thrombosis is similar in BMS and DES. On the other hand, late (1 month–1 year) and very late (beyond 1 year) stent thrombosis is more frequent and occurs almost exclusively in DES because of delayed arterial healing and poor endothelialization, particularly when implanted for off-label indications, including left main, bypass grafts, AMI, and bifurcation lesions compared with on-label indications.[21] We compared DES lesions with late thrombosis with those without thrombosis to determine the best predictor of late stent thrombosis; poor endothelialization that correlated with the ratio of uncovered to total stent struts per section on histology was the best predictor of late stent thrombosis. By multivariate analysis, the presence of more than 30% uncovered stent struts was associated with a 9 times greater chance of late stent thrombosis.[22]

The delayed healing in DES is also influenced by the underlying plaque morphology. For example, patients with DES implanted for acute plaque rupture had greater delayed arterial healing (ie, uncovered struts, less neointimal thickness, inflammation, and fibrin deposition) compared with those with stable plaque (**Fig. 3**). The delayed healing was also greater at rupture sites versus non-rupture sites within the same stent (proximal and distal). Furthermore, we have observed a significantly higher incidence of late stent thrombosis in patients treated for plaque rupture compared with those with stable lesions, which emphasizes the importance of the underlying plaque morphology in arterial healing after DES implantation.[23]

### Hypersensitivity Reactions in DES

Virmani and colleagues[24] were the first to report a case of hypersensitivity reaction in DES, which is a rare but important complication after DES implantation. It is sometimes accompanied by

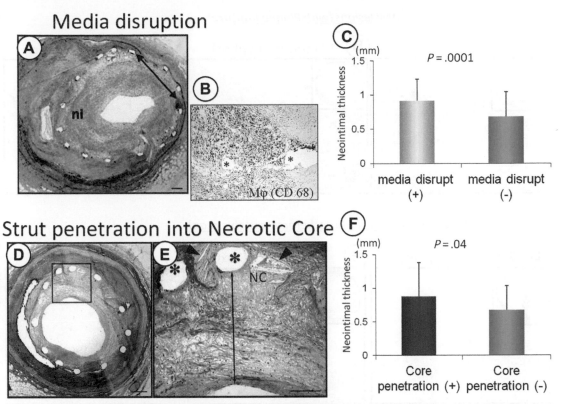

**Fig. 2.** Media injury and necrotic core penetration by stent struts increase the risk of restenosis in BMS. Photomicrograph (*A*) showing the association of arterial injury (medial disruption, *arrow* in *A*) with increased neointimal (ni) thickness. CD68 immunohistochemistry (*B*) identifies numerous brown-staining macrophages around struts (*asterisks*). Bar graph (*C*) showing greater neointimal thickness above struts with media injury compared with those without media injury. Necrotic core (NC) penetration by stent struts (low power in *D* and high power in *E*) was associated with increased neointimal thickness (*arrow*). Cholesterol clefts are indicated by *arrowheads* in *E*. Bar graph (*F*) shows increased neointimal thickness above the struts with necrotic core penetration compared with those without necrotic core penetration. (*Modified and reproduced from* Farb A, Weber DK, Kolodgie FD, et al. Morphologic predictors of restenosis after coronary stenting in humans. Circulation 2002;105(25):2976–8; with permission.)

systemic manifestations including rash, itching, hives, or dyspnea[25]; however, these symptoms are not always present because hypersensitivity can be limited to the localized area of the stent. Histologically, hypersensitivity reaction is characterized by extensive inflammatory cell infiltration of the vessel walls, consisting of eosinophils and lymphocytes, with multinuclear giant cells seen close to the stent struts and polymer (**Fig. 4**). The inflammation is associated with positive remodeling of the vessel, resulting in malapposition and subsequently late stent thrombosis. If multiple Cypher (Cordis, Bridgewater, NJ, USA) sirolimus-eluting stents (SES) are placed in the same individual, all SES are involved by hypersensitivity irrespective of location, suggesting the existence of a localized immunologic reaction. In our DES registry, hypersensitivity reaction is exclusively observed in SES.[22] Because most of the cases with hypersensitivity reaction have been seen beyond the 1-year period, it is more likely related to the polymer rather than sirolimus, because the drug is expected to be completely eluted by this time. The characteristic appearance of the granulomatous tissue in optical coherence tomography consists of dark signal intensity and a heterogeneous texture, along with the scalloped appearance of the lumen.[26]

### Neoatherosclerosis Within In-stent Area

Neoatherosclerosis is defined as newly formed atherosclerotic change within the in-stent area. Neoatherosclerosis at the site of BMS implantation is rarely reported and usually occurs beyond 5 years. However, we have reported a case of

*AMI lesions (with Plaque Rupture)*

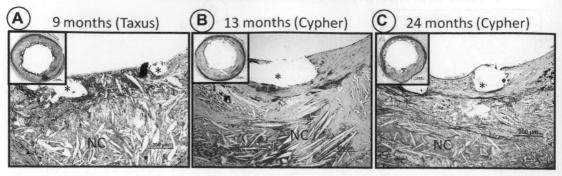

*Stable Lesions (with Fibroatheroma and thick cap)*

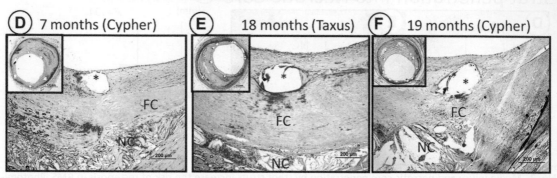

**Fig. 3.** Vascular healing after DES implantation for the treatment of AMI or stable angina. (*A–C*) Histologic sections from patients with AMI: a 64-year-old woman who died of congestive heart failure 9 months after Taxus stent implantation (*A*), a 49-year-old man who died of noncardiac cause 13 months after Cypher stent implantation (*B*), and a 34-year-old woman who died of late stent thrombosis 24 months after Cypher stent implantation (*C*). Struts with necrotic core (NC) were observed with fibrin deposition and the absence of endothelial coverage (*A*). Stents in *B* and *C* showed minimal coverage of struts above the necrotic core at 13 and 24 months. (*D–F*) Histologic sections from patients with stable lesions: a 61-year-old man who died of a noncardiac cause 7 months after Cypher stent implantation (*D*), a 53-year-old man who died suddenly 18 months after Taxus stent implantation (*E*), and a 68-year-old man who died of a noncardiac cause 19 months after Cypher stent implantation (*F*). All patients had underlying fibroatheroma with thick fibrous cap (FC). High-magnification images show underlying necrotic core and a thick fibrous cap with various degrees of neointimal formation above the stent struts (*D–F*). (*Reproduced from* Nakazawa G, Finn AV, Joner M, et al. Delayed arterial healing and increased late stent thrombosis at culprit sites after drug-eluting stent placement for acute myocardial infarction patients: an autopsy study. Circulation 2008;118(11):1143; with permission.)

sudden death caused by plaque rupture within the stented segment 9 years after implantation.[27] Therefore, late symptoms in patients receiving BMS may be related to advanced atherosclerotic changes within the neointima.[28] Recently, we reviewed our cases from our BMS and DES registry for lesions with neoatherosclerosis, which is represented by the presence of lipid-laden foamy macrophages with or without necrotic core formation, without communicating with the underlying atherosclerotic plaque. The incidence of neoatherosclerosis was significantly greater in DES (35%) than BMS (10%) in stent implants more than 3 months and less than 60 months. Furthermore, there was a substantial difference in the timing of neoatherosclerosis, with the earliest changes in BMS being observed beyond 2 years, and at 4 months for DES. Thus, rapid neoatherosclerotic change observed in DES suggests the possibility that late thrombotic events in DES could be related to accelerated neoatherosclerosis.[29]

## Gender Difference of Stenting in Patients with ACS

To investigate the gender difference in stenting in patients with ACS, we examined 118 coronary segments from patients (25 lesions from women, 93 lesions from men) with DES (SES, n = 52; paclitaxel-eluting stents, n = 49; zotalimus-eluting

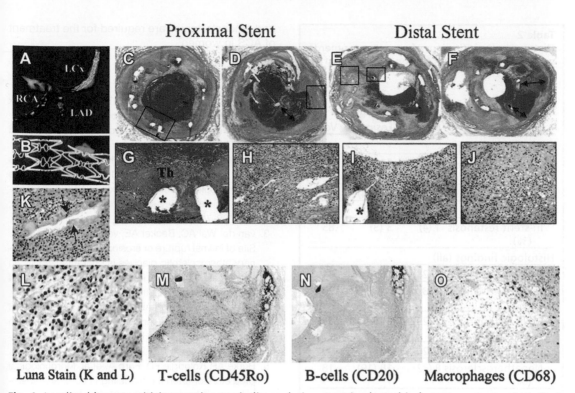

**Fig. 4.** Localized hypersensitivity reaction to sirolimus-eluting stent implanted in human coronary artery. Post-mortem radiographs (*A, B*) showing 2 LCx Cypher stents; note absence of stent overlap (*B*). Photomicrographs of representative cross-sections of proximal (*C, D*) and distal (*E, F*) Cypher stents. Focal strut malapposition with aneurysmal dilatation (*double arrows* in *D* and *F*) and occlusive luminal thrombosis (Th, *C* and *D*) are present. (*G–J*) High-power views of stented artery from proximal (*C, D*) and distal (*E*) boxed areas. (*G*) Luminal thrombus (Th) above stent struts with absence of SMC. There is diffuse inflammation within intima and media (*H, boxed area* in *D*). (*I*) (*Right box* in *E*) Extensive inflammation consisting primarily of eosinophils and lymphocytes, with a focal giant cell reaction around stent strut (*asterisks*) and surrounding polymer. Marked inflammation is similarly present in intima, media, and adventitia in *J* (*left box* in *E*). (*K, L*) Luna stains show giant cells (*arrowheads*) around a polymer remnant that has separated from the stent strut and numerous eosinophils within the arterial wall. (*M–O*) Immunohistochemical identification of T cells (CD45Ro), B cells (CD20), and macrophages (CD68), respectively; T lymphocytes are the predominant inflammatory cell type. (*Reproduced from* Virmani R, Guagliumi G, Farb A, et al. Localized hypersensitivity and late coronary thrombosis secondary to a sirolimus-eluting stent: should we be cautious? Circulation 2004;109(6):703; with permission.)

stents, n = 5; everolimus-eluting stents, n = 13) implanted for the treatment of ACS in which the underlying plaque morphology was remarkably divergent between men and women; plaque rupture (necrotic core prolapse) was more frequently observed in men (38%) than in women (16%) (*P* = .041) (**Table 2**). On the contrary, pathologic intimal thickening (PIT) was the predominant morphologic finding in women (32%), whereas in men PIT was the underlying plaque in ACS in only 10% of lesions. These results are in concordance with the earlier discussion regarding plaque rupture and erosion, because the underlying mechanism of ACS between men and women is different.

The incidence of restenosis, which was defined as more than 75% cross-sectional area luminal narrowing within the stent, was significantly higher in women than in men (20% vs 4%, respectively, *P* = .001). There was a higher rate of mild eosinophil infiltration in women than in men (20% vs 6%, respectively, *P* = .039), whereas there was no significant difference in the occurrence of other pathologic changes such as thrombosis, hypersensitivity, and neoatherosclerosis within the stent segments. Although the precise cause of the discrepancies between men and women remains unknown, a plausible explanation might include small vessel size and vasospasm in women that would lead to greater injury and subsequent inflammation within stented regions; moreover, there may be gender differences in susceptibility to antiproliferative drugs or polymers; thrombus burden or degree of healing (thrombus age) at the time of intervention may also be involved.

**Table 2**
**Histopathologic findings of coronary segments with DES implantation for the treatment of ACS**

| | Women (n = 25 Lesions) | Men (n = 93 Lesions) | P Value |
|---|---|---|---|
| Underlying disease | | | |
| Plaque rupture (%) | 4 (16) | 35 (38) | .041 |
| TCFA (%) | 4 (16) | 22 (24) | .41 |
| PIT (%) | 8 (32) | 9 (10) | .005 |
| In-stent restenosis (%) | 1 (4) | 3 (3) | .85 |
| Histologic findings (all) | | | |
| Thrombosis (%) | 7 (28) | 28 (30) | .84 |
| Hypersensitivity (%) | 2 (8) | 3 (3) | .29 |
| Mild eosinophil infiltration (%) | 5 (20) | 6 (6) | .039 |
| Restenosis (%) | 5 (20) | 4 (4) | .001 |
| Neoatherosclerosis (%) | 8 (32) | 18 (19) | .18 |
| Histologic findings (<30 d) | | | |
| Thrombosis (%) | 3/10 (30) | 11/37 (30) | .99 |
| Histologic findings (>30 d) | | | |
| Thrombosis (%) | 4/15 (27) | 17/56 (30) | .78 |
| Hypersensitivity (%) | 2/15 (13) | 2/56 (4) | .15 |
| Mild eosinophil infiltration (%) | 4/15 (27) | 5/56 (9) | .067 |
| Restenosis (%) | 5/15 (33) | 4/56 (7) | .007 |
| Neoatherosclerosis (%) | 7/15 (47) | 18/56 (32) | .30 |

Values correspond to the number of lesions; those in parentheses are percentages.

Further investigations are required to elucidate these differences.

## Summary

Autopsy studies have revealed distinct evidence of gender difference in the cause and pathogenesis underlying ACS events in which plaque rupture is more common in men and erosion in women, with the latter being the predominate lesion in women presenting with ACS. Our study showed that the prevailing strategy of treatment of patients with ACS by stenting regardless of the underlying plaque morphology leads to a higher rate of restenosis in women than in men. Therefore stenting may not be an appropriate therapy in women,

and other strategies are required for the treatment of ACS in women.

## REFERENCES

1. Burke AP, Farb A, Malcom GT, et al. Coronary risk factors and plaque morphology in men with coronary disease who died suddenly. N Engl J Med 1997;336:1276–82.
2. Virmani R, Kolodgie FD, Burke AP, et al. Lessons from sudden coronary death: a comprehensive morphological classification scheme for atherosclerotic lesions. Arterioscler Thromb Vasc Biol 2000; 20:1262–75.
3. van der Wal AC, Becker AE, van der Loos CM, et al. Site of intimal rupture or erosion of thrombosed coronary atherosclerotic plaques is characterized by an inflammatory process irrespective of the dominant plaque morphology. Circulation 1994;89:36–44.
4. Kolodgie FD, Burke AP, Farb A, et al. Differential accumulation of proteoglycans and hyaluronan in culprit lesions: insights into plaque erosion. Arterioscler Thromb Vasc Biol 2002;22:1642–8.
5. Burke AP, Kolodgie FD, Farb A, et al. Morphological predictors of arterial remodeling in coronary atherosclerosis. Circulation 2002;105:297–303.
6. Hao H, Gabbiani G, Camenzind E, et al. Phenotypic modulation of intima and media smooth muscle cells in fatal cases of coronary artery lesion. Arterioscler Thromb Vasc Biol 2006;26:326–32.
7. Kramer MC, Rittersma SZ, de Winter RJ, et al. Relationship of thrombus healing to underlying plaque morphology in sudden coronary death. J Am Coll Cardiol 2010;55:122–32.
8. Kramer MC, van der Wal AC, Koch KT, et al. Presence of older thrombus is an independent predictor of long-term mortality in patients with ST-elevation myocardial infarction treated with thrombus aspiration during primary percutaneous coronary intervention. Circulation 2008;118:1810–6.
9. Kannel WB, Schatzkin A. Sudden death: lessons from subsets in population studies. J Am Coll Cardiol 1985;5:141B–9B.
10. Arbustini E, Dal Bello B, Morbini P, et al. Plaque erosion is a major substrate for coronary thrombosis in acute myocardial infarction. Heart 1999; 82:269–72.
11. Burke AP, Farb A, Malcom GT, et al. Effect of risk factors on the mechanism of acute thrombosis and sudden coronary death in women. Circulation 1998;97:2110–6.
12. Adams MR, Williams JK, Clarkson TB, et al. Effects of oestrogens and progestogens on coronary atherosclerosis and osteoporosis of monkeys. Baillieres Clin Obstet Gynaecol 1991;5:915–34.
13. Foegh ML, Zhao Y, Farhat M, et al. Oestradiol inhibition of vascular myointimal proliferation following

immune, chemical and mechanical injury. Ciba Found Symp 1995;191:139–45 [discussion: 145–9].

14. Ouyang P, Michos ED, Karas RH. Hormone replacement therapy and the cardiovascular system lessons learned and unanswered questions. J Am Coll Cardiol 2006;47:1741–53.

15. Farb A, Sangiorgi G, Carter AJ, et al. Pathology of acute and chronic coronary stenting in humans. Circulation 1999;99:44–52.

16. Virmani R, Farb A. Pathology of in-stent restenosis. Curr Opin Lipidol 1999;10:499–506.

17. Komatsu R, Ueda M, Naruko T, et al. Neointimal tissue response at sites of coronary stenting in humans: macroscopic, histological, and immunohistochemical analyses. Circulation 1998;98:224–33.

18. Schwartz SM, deBlois D, O'Brien ER. The intima. Soil for atherosclerosis and restenosis. Circ Res 1995; 77:445–65.

19. Topol EJ, Serruys PW. Frontiers in interventional cardiology. Circulation 1998;98:1802–20.

20. Farb A, Weber DK, Kolodgie FD, et al. Morphological predictors of restenosis after coronary stenting in humans. Circulation 2002;105:2974–80.

21. Kaul S, Shah PK, Diamond GA. As time goes by: current status and future directions in the controversy over stenting. J Am Coll Cardiol 2007;50:128–37.

22. Finn AV, Joner M, Nakazawa G, et al. Pathological correlates of late drug-eluting stent thrombosis: strut coverage as a marker of endothelialization. Circulation 2007;115:2435–41.

23. Nakazawa G, Finn AV, Joner M, et al. Delayed arterial healing and increased late stent thrombosis at culprit sites after drug-eluting stent placement for acute myocardial infarction patients: an autopsy study. Circulation 2008;118:1138–45.

24. Virmani R, Guagliumi G, Farb A, et al. Localized hypersensitivity and late coronary thrombosis secondary to a sirolimus-eluting stent: should we be cautious? Circulation 2004;109:701–5.

25. Nebeker JR, Virmani R, Bennett CL, et al. Hypersensitivity cases associated with drug-eluting coronary stents: a review of available cases from the research on adverse drug events and reports (radar) project. J Am Coll Cardiol 2006;47:175–81.

26. Sawada T, Shite J, Shinke T, et al. Very late thrombosis of sirolimus-eluting stent due to late malapposition: serial observations with optical coherence tomography. J Cardiol 2008;52:290–5.

27. Ramcharitar S, Hochadel M, Gaster AL, et al. An insight into the current use of drug eluting stents in acute and elective percutaneous coronary interventions in Europe. A report on the EuroPCI Survey. EuroIntervention 2008;3:429–41.

28. Chen MS, John JM, Chew DP, et al. Bare metal stent restenosis is not a benign clinical entity. Am Heart J 2006;151:1260–4.

29. Nakazawa G, Otsuka F, Nakano M, et al. The pathology of neoatherosclerosis in human coronary implants bare-metal and drug-eluting stents. J Am Coll Cardiol 2011;57:1314–22.

# Does Gender have an Influence on Platelet Function and the Efficacy of Oral Antiplatelet Therapy?

Udaya S. Tantry, PhD[a], Eliano P. Navarese, MD[b],
Paul A. Gurbel, MD[a],*

**KEYWORDS**

- Antiplatelet therapy • Platelet function • Thrombogenicity
- Gender difference

The underlying pathophysiology of ischemic complications during acute coronary syndrome (ACS) involves thrombus generation at sites of plaque rupture and endothelial erosion. Platelet activation and aggregation play major roles in the latter process. Following plaque rupture, platelet adhesion to exposed collagen and von Willebrand factor by specific receptors and the binding of thrombin generated by tissue factor to protease-activated receptors (PARs) cause platelet activation. Subsequently, adenosine diphosphate (ADP) is released from dense granules; platelet cyclooxygenase-1 (COX-1) converts arachidonic acid (originating from membrane phospholipids) to prostaglandin (PG)$H_2$; and platelet-specific thromboxane (Tx) synthase converts $PGH_2$ to $TxA_2$, which is released from activated platelets. By autocrine and paracrine mechanisms, these agonists are responsible for the amplification of platelet activation and aggregation.[1] Most importantly, continuous ADP-$P2Y_{12}$ receptor signaling is essential for the sustained activation of the GPIIb/IIIa receptor and stable thrombus generation. Simultaneously, platelet activation exposes the phosphatidylserine surface, providing binding sites for coagulation factors and the generation of thrombin. The fibrin network generated by thrombin activity binds to the aggregated platelets and forms the stable platelet fibrin clot at the site of vascular injury.[1]

Currently approved antiplatelet strategies for secondary prevention in patients with ACS include inhibition of COX-1 by aspirin, inhibition of the ADP-$P2Y_{12}$ interaction by $P2Y_{12}$ receptor antagonists, and inhibition of the GPIIb/IIIa receptor by GPIIb/IIIa inhibitors.[2] Aspirin is the bedrock of antiplatelet treatment strategies, for primary as well as secondary prevention. In the Women's Health Study (n = 39,876), a primary prevention study, there was a significant benefit of aspirin therapy in reducing stroke (risk ratio = 0.83, 95% confidence interval = 0.69–0.99) but no benefit in reducing combined cardiovascular events, myocardial infarction (MI), and death.[3] The earlier meta-analysis of 6 primary prevention trials (n= ~70,000 high-risk vascular disease patients) by the Antithrombotic Trialists' (ATT) collaboration reported a 12% reduction in serious vascular events, mainly attributable to a 20% reduction in nonfatal MI, and no differences in the reduction of specific vascular outcomes based on gender

Dr Gurbel received research grants, honoraria, and consultant fees from Hemonetics, AstraZeneca, Merck, Medtronic, Lilly/Daiichi Sankyo, Sanofi Aventis/Bristol Myers, Boston-Scientific, Bayer, Novartis, Accumetrics, Boehringer Ingelheim, and Johnson and Johnson. Dr Tantry and Dr Navarese report no conflict of interest.

[a] Cardiac Catheterization Laboratory, Sinai Center for Thrombosis Research, 2401 West Belvedere Avenue, Baltimore, MD 21215, USA
[b] Interventional Cardio-Angiology Unit, GVM Care and Research, Cotignola, Ravenna, Italy
* Corresponding author.
E-mail address: PGURBEL@LIFEBRIDGEHEALTH.ORG

Intervent Cardiol Clin 1 (2012) 223–230
doi:10.1016/j.iccl.2012.01.007
2211-7458/12/$ – see front matter © 2012 Elsevier Inc. All rights reserved.

after adjustment for multiple comparisons.[4] In a subsequent gender-specific meta-analysis based on 6 trials with a total of 95,456 individuals; 3 trials included only men, 1 included only women, and 2 included both sexes, Berger and colleagues[5] reported a significant 12% ($P$ = .03) reduction in cardiovascular events associated with aspirin therapy among women (n = 51,342) that was driven mainly by a significant 17% reduction in ischemic stroke ($P$ = .02). In the recent ATT analysis, there was a borderline influence of gender on the effect of aspirin; men derived a greater benefit for the primary prevention of major coronary events. Although there were no differences in the beneficial effect of aspirin on serious vascular event occurrence between genders in primary prevention, aspirin therapy was more effective in reducing ischemic stroke among women and major coronary event occurrence among men, with a $P$ = .08 for heterogeneity (**Fig. 1**A). For secondary prevention among women, aspirin therapy was more effective in reducing major coronary events but was not effective in reducing ischemic stroke. The influence of gender ($P$ for heterogeneity) for secondary prevention was not significant for any outcomes (see **Fig. 1**B).[6]

Meta-analysis of large-scale clinical studies including a wide spectrum of patients (n = 79,624) with coronary artery disease (CAD) demonstrated that therapy with aspirin and clopidogrel is associated with a significant reduction in ischemic event occurrence compared with aspirin therapy alone.[7] In another gender-specific meta-analysis of these trials (n = 79,613), no definite influence of gender on clinical outcomes was reported. However, among women (n = 23,533) the risk reduction with clopidogrel therapy appeared greatest for MI (18% reduction); the effects on stroke and cardiovascular death were not significant (9% and 1% reductions, respectively). In men (n = 56,091) there was a significant reduction in MI, stroke, and total death associated with clopidogrel therapy (16%, 17%, and 17% reductions, respectively). Adding clopidogrel to aspirin resulted in a 43% versus a 22% increased rate of major bleeding in women and men, respectively.[8]

In an analysis of the Clopidogrel for High Atherothrombotic Risk and Ischemic Stabilization, Management, and Avoidance (CHARISMA) trial, there appeared to be a trend for better outcome among men than among women treated with clopidogrel.[9] In the Clopidogrel and Aspirin Optimal Dose Usage to Reduce Recurrent Events–Seventh Organization to Assess Strategies in Ischemic Syndromes (CURRENT OASIS 7) trial, there was a higher event rate among women (4.1% double/

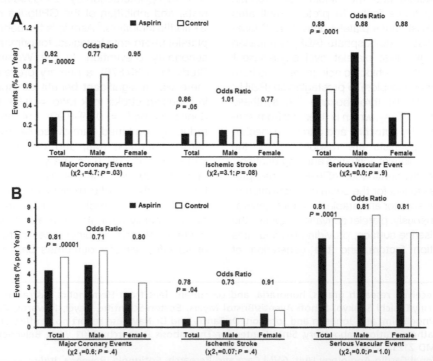

**Fig. 1.** (*A*) Yearly event rates in primary prevention trials with respect to gender. (*B*) Yearly event rates in secondary prevention trials with respect to gender. (*Data from* Antithrombotic Trialists' (ATT) Collaboration, Baigent C, Blackwell L, Collins R, et al. Aspirin in the primary and secondary prevention of vascular disease: collaborative meta-analysis of individual participant data from randomised trials. Lancet 2009;373:1849–60.)

4.1% standard clopidogrel [men] versus 4.5% double/5.4% standard clopidogrel [women]; P for interaction = 0.17) in both standard and double-dose clopidogrel-treated patients.[10] In the trial to assess improvement in therapeutic outcomes by optimizing platelet inhibition with prasugrel—Thrombolysis in Myocardial Infarction (TRITON-TIMI) 38 trial, women had a higher rate of primary end-point occurrence in both clopidogrel-treated and prasugrel-treated groups (11.9% [clopidogrel] vs 9.5% [prasugrel] in men and 12.6% [clopidogrel] vs 11.0% [prasugrel] in women, respectively), and prasugrel therapy was numerically less effective in women (risk reduction = 21% in men vs 12% in women).[11] Moreover, female gender was associated with a significantly increased hazard ratio for non–coronary artery bypass graft–related events in an independent Cox regression analysis (hazard ratio = 1.77, P<.001, strength of association with bleeding = 28.79).[12] In the Platelet Inhibition and Patient Outcome (PLATO) trial, there were no differences in efficacy associated with clopidogrel and ticagrelor therapy between men and women (P for interaction = 0.82), but women had a numerically increased rate of primary end-point occurrence (men = 11.1% [clopidogrel] vs 9.2% [ticagrelor]; women = 13.2% [clopidogrel] vs 11.2% [ticagrelor]).[13] The latter recent trials indicate that female gender tends to be associated with an increased rate of primary end-point occurrence irrespective of $P2Y_{12}$ receptor therapy. Whether higher platelet reactivity or a diminished antiplatelet response among women plays a role in this observation is unknown.

The relative delay in the onset of ischemic heart disease in women compared with men has been attributed to vascular protection by premenopausal estrogen production. However, there is limited basic, epidemiologic, or clinical evidence to firmly support this theory.[14,15] A recent modeling study including proportional age-related changes in ischemic heart disease data from England, Wales, and the United States demonstrated an exponential increase in heart disease mortality in women throughout all ages without any specific increase at menopausal ages; there was a greater increase in mortality from heart disease during early adulthood in men than in women, and the age-related increment in heart disease mortality was blunted at advanced age in men.[16]

## GENDER-RELATED DIFFERENCE IN PLATELET REACTIVITY
### Animal Studies

Cardiovascular diseases are more frequent in men than in premenopausal women, and are similar in postmenopausal women and men of the similar age. Conversely, use of oral contraceptives was associated with an increase in the incidence of thromboembolic disease.[17] It was postulated that estrogen has a protective influence on the cardio-vascular system including a beneficial effect on platelet function. However, an increase as well as attenuation in platelet response induced by estrogens has been reported in rats.[18,19]

In an in vivo experimental model of thrombosis, male rats showed increased thrombus formation when compared with female rats. In female rats, thrombus formation was influenced by the estrous cycle, with an enhanced thrombus deposition during the diestrus stage. Treatment with the synthetic estrogen, ethinyl estradiol, for 6 weeks was associated with a significantly reduced thrombus deposition in both male and female rats, which was dependent on the concentration of heparin used.[20] In a subsequent in vitro experiment by the same group, platelets isolated from female and male rats were equally responsive to adenosine diphosphate (ADP), collagen, and arachidonic acid, indicating similar intrinsic platelet reactivity, whereas platelets isolated from male rats were less sensitive to thrombin and more sensitive to inhibition by prostaglandin $I_2$ than those from females. There were no differences in the coagulation parameters, activated partial thromboplastin time, and prothrombin time between male and female rats, but fibrinogen levels were almost 2 times higher in male rat plasma. Following 6 weeks of 17β-estradiol or ethinyl estradiol treatment in female rats, no effect on ADP-, arachidonic acid-, thrombin-, or collagen-induced platelet aggregation was observed but there was a reduction in adenosine triphosphate (ATP) release induced by collagen, which the investigators suggested to be responsible for inhibition of thrombus formation in female rats observed in the earlier in vivo experiments. Furthermore, the investigators suggested that increased fibrinogen levels in male rats may contribute to the increased thrombus formation in male rats.[20]

In another rat thrombosis model, thrombus size and mortality rate were twice as high in male rats than in female rats and were exacerbated by testosterone in both genders, but estradiol decreased thrombus weight in male rats only. Anti-androgen treatment with flutamide significantly reduced the mortality rate in both genders treated with testosterone.[21,22] Johnson and colleagues[23] demonstrated that platelet responsiveness to ADP was 10 times higher in male rats than in female rats; castration significantly reduced platelet response to ADP in male rats, but ovariectomy enhanced responsiveness in female rats.

Testosterone treatment in physiologic concentrations consistently enhanced platelet response in both sexes and also restored the reduced platelet response in castrated male rats. Furthermore, platelet response was enhanced by incubation of platelets isolated from rats and guinea pigs with testosterone.[22] In vivo treatment of estradiol, as well as in vitro incubation of estradiol, progesterone, and deoxycorticosterone, showed an inhibitory effect on platelet response. The enhanced platelet response with testosterone demonstrated in in vitro experiments was antagonized by flutamide and also by estradiol.[23]

Leng and colleagues[24] demonstrated that platelets isolated from female mice compared with those from male mice demonstrated a higher tendency to bind to fibrinogen in response to low concentrations of thrombin and collagen-related peptide (CRP), and greater aggregation in response to ADP and CRP. Moreover, they demonstrated that these properties were intrinsic to platelets, because they were observed in washed platelets but not when platelets were present in plasma.

Male dogs showed a greater maximal contractile response to U46619 and greater sensitivity (lower $EC_{50}$) of coronary and renal vessels, which was reduced significantly by estrogen treatment.[25] Testosterone has been shown to upregulate platelet thromboxane $A_2$ receptor expression and enhance platelet response to $TxA_2$ mimetic U46619. In another experiment, male diabetic Zucker rats showed an impaired response to vasoconstrictors (U46619 and angiotensin-II) and to endothelial (NO)-mediated vasodilation, which may be related to the greater prothrombotic activity and a worse impairment of endothelial reactivity in the type-2 diabetic state.[26] Thus, overall, testosterone seems to enhance the platelet response to agonists and has prothrombotic properties, whereas estrogen seems to overcome these prothrombotic properties.

## GENDER-RELATED DIFFERENCE IN PLATELET REACTIVITY
### Human Studies

In a case-control study of 53 men with coronary heart disease younger than 50 years and in 48 control subjects without coronary heart disease who were matched for age, sex, and socioeconomic status, it was observed that patients with coronary heart disease showed significantly increased mean platelet volume, and greater adrenaline-induced but not ADP- or collagen-induced platelet aggregation, which was weakly ($r = -0.28$, $P<.05$) associated with the severity of CAD lesions but not the extent of the disease. This finding suggests that platelets play a role in the development of plaque progression and thrombosis at the site of plaque rupture.[27] In a study by Kurrelmeyer and colleagues[28] involving 400 asymptomatic men and women with a family history of premature coronary artery disease, platelets from women showed increased fibrinogen binding in response to ADP and greater spontaneous aggregation compared with platelets from men. In the same study, women had higher levels of plasma thromboxane $B_2$ levels compared with men.

Yee and colleagues[29] demonstrated that a minority of healthy volunteers showed hyperresponsiveness ($\geq 65\%$ maximal platelet aggregation) to ADP, collagen, epinephrine, CRP, and ristocetin; female gender and higher fibrinogen levels were strongly associated with hyperresponsiveness. In the population-based cohort study in the Molise region of Italy involving 18,907 subjects, women had significantly higher platelet indices such as platelet count, plateletcrit, and mean platelet volume. Moreover, platelet count and plateletcrit were positively associated with inflammation indices such as white blood cell count, C-reactive protein levels, and D-dimer levels. In addition, the investigators demonstrated that the difference in platelet indices between men and women persisted at any age range and also after menopause.[30] In another study involving 958 participants, platelet aggregation in response to ADP was higher in women than in men, and there was a strong relation between plasma fibrinogen concentration and platelet reactivity. Based on these data, the investigators suggested that hormonal influences may be responsible.[31] In another study in the absence of antiplatelet therapy, platelets from women were more reactive to multiple agonists in comparison with men.[32] In addition, it has been reported that the number of activated GPIIb/IIIa receptors per platelet capable of binding fibrinogen or PAC-1 in response to ADP and thrombin receptor–activating peptide was significantly higher in women than in men; however, no differences in the total number of GPIIb/IIIa receptor expression was observed. Based on these observations, the investigators suggested that platelet GPIIb/IIIa receptors in premenopausal women are more activatable than platelet GPIIb/IIIa receptors in young men, and that hormonal variations may modulate GPIIb/IIIa expression.[33]

It was demonstrated in postmenopausal women that estrogens reduce thromboxane $B_2$ production, and that estrogen replacement therapy reduces ex vivo platelet aggregation and ATP release in response to ADP.[34] In vitro exposure of platelets to 17β-estradiol has been shown to inhibit ADP-induced platelet aggregation and ATP release.[35] It has also been shown that platelets from both men and women express estrogen receptors and receptor-associated proteins. The aforementioned effects of estrogen may be mediated by platelet estrogen receptors.[36] It has been demonstrated that estrogen influences proplatelet formation and platelet production. In addition, continuous estrogen therapy has been shown to decrease plasma concentrations of fibrinogen, antithrombin, protein S, and plasminogen activator inhibitor.[37]

## ANTIPLATELET RESPONSE TO ASPIRIN IN WOMEN

In 1985, Harrison and Weisblatt[38] demonstrated that spontaneous platelet aggregation but not collagen-induced aggregation was inhibited by the in vitro addition of aspirin (40 μg/mL) to platelets from men but not from women. This inhibitory effect was reduced in orchiectomized male patients and was restored by adding testosterone but not estradiol. The investigators suggested that higher levels of COX activity caused by (1) higher concentrations of testosterone in men, (2) less effectiveness of aspirin in acetylating COX in women, or (3) gender-dependent effects of aspirin that are independent of COX-1 inhibition may explain the attenuated effect of aspirin in women.[39] In support of the latter non–COX-1 effects of aspirin, greater inhibition of thrombus formation in male rats and ex vivo thrombus generation in a Baumgartner chamber with blood isolated from men were demonstrated in the presence of complete inhibition of COX-1 in both genders by aspirin.[40,41]

Becker and colleagues[32] studied platelet reactivity in healthy subjects who were siblings of patients with documented coronary heart disease, and showed in women a significantly higher platelet reactivity to multiple agonists compared with men, in the absence of antiplatelet therapy. Following 81-mg aspirin therapy for 14 days, platelets from women had a consistently greater response to multiple agonists, and the latter effect was more pronounced in laboratory assays that were indirectly dependent on COX-1 activity. In COX-1–specific assays, aspirin therapy was associated with similar and near total suppression of residual platelet aggregation in both men and women. However, there was a modest increase in residual platelet reactivity in women compared with men, regardless of age. Baseline platelet function contributed most to the variance in aggregation after aspirin therapy.[32] The same investigators further studied the antiplatelet effect of 14 days' therapy with 81 mg/d and 325 mg/d aspirin

in 106 healthy volunteers who were siblings of patients with documented coronary heart disease.[42] The investigators again showed that the differences in platelet reactivity between men and women became more evident after aspirin therapy, and there was a lower inhibitory effect in women that persisted even after 325 mg/d therapy. Based on impedance aggregometry in diluted whole blood, Ivandic and colleagues[43] measured the antiplatelet response to aspirin using collagen and arachidonic acid in healthy subjects and patients with CAD. A significantly stronger collagen-induced platelet aggregation was observed among healthy women compared with healthy men, which persisted even after in vitro sample incubation with aspirin or terbogrel (a combined inhibitor of thromboxane synthase and thromboxane receptor). Among CAD patients, women showed a stronger collagen-induced platelet aggregation than did men during aspirin therapy, but not during aspirin and clopidogrel therapy.

## ANTIPLATELET RESPONSE TO ASPIRIN AND CLOPIDOGREL IN WOMEN

Clopidogrel is metabolized by hepatic cytochromes into an active metabolite that irreversibly inhibits the platelet P2Y$_{12}$ receptor. It has been shown that women have higher cytochrome (CYP) 2C19 and CYP3A4 activity. These cytochromes are important in clopidogrel metabolism.[44,45] However, the influence of single-nucleotide polymorphisms on clopidogrel metabolism, pharmacodynamics, and clinical efficacy in relation to gender has not been demonstrated. In a recent genome-wide association study conducted in a healthy Amish population, gender was modestly associated with clopidogrel response, with women tending to respond less well than men. Differences in antiplatelet response to more potent P2Y$_{12}$ receptor blockers such as prasugrel and ticagrelor with respect to gender have not been evaluated.[46]

It has been shown that race and gender play significant roles in thrombogenicity in patients treated with stenting (n = 252). Adverse ischemic events 6 months after stenting were higher in women, and African Americans had higher event rates than Caucasians. The highest event rates were observed in African American women and the lowest in African American men. Thrombogenicity as measured by thrombin-induced platelet-fibrin clot strength was greatest in African American women (**Fig. 2**). In a multivariate logistic regression analysis, platelet fibrin clot strength (relative risk = 2.52, $P = .017$) and gender (relative risk = 2.56, $P = .009$) were significant independent predictors of 6-month adverse event occurrence (see **Fig. 2**).[47]

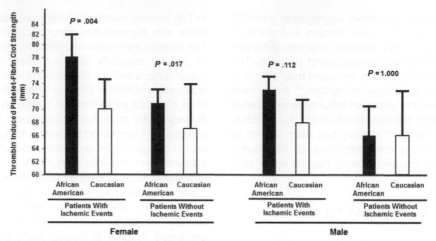

**Fig. 2.** Thrombin-induced platelet fibrin clot strength in patients with and without ischemic event occurrence with respect to race and gender. (*Data from* Gurbel PA, Bliden KP, Cohen E, et al. Race and sex differences in thrombogenicity: risk of ischemic events following coronary stenting. Blood Coagul Fibrinolysis 2008;19:268–75.)

## SUMMARY

At this time it remains speculative whether there are intrinsic differences in thrombogenicity between genders. In contemporary trials of ACS with dual antiplatelet therapy strategies, women tend to experience greater rates of ischemic events. Controversy exists surrounding the protective role of estrogens in the premenopausal woman. In vitro studies support the attenuation of platelet function by estrogen. The mechanisms behind this observation remain uncertain. However, there is enough provocative data supporting the presence of gender differences in thrombogenicity to promote further investigation in this exciting area.

## REFERENCES

1. Gurbel PA, Bliden KP, Hayes KM, et al. Platelet activation in myocardial ischemic syndromes. Expert Rev Cardiovasc Ther 2004;2:535–45.
2. Wright RS, Anderson JL, Adams CD, et al. 2011 ACCF/AHA Focused Update of the Guidelines for the Management of Patients With Unstable Angina/Non-ST-Elevation Myocardial Infarction (Updating the 2007 Guideline) A report of the American College of Cardiology Foundation/American Heart Association Task Force on Practice Guidelines. J Am Coll Cardiol 2011;57:e215–367.
3. Ridker PM, Cook NR, Lee IM, et al. A randomized trial of low-dose aspirin in the primary prevention of cardiovascular disease in women. N Engl J Med 2005;352:1293–304.
4. Antithrombotic Trialists' Collaboration. Collaborative meta-analysis of randomised trials of antiplatelet therapy for prevention of death, myocardial infarction, and stroke in high risk patients. BMJ 2002;324:71–86.
5. Berger JS, Roncaglioni MC, Avanzini F, et al. Aspirin for the primary prevention of cardiovascular events in women and men: a sex-specific meta-analysis of randomized controlled trials. JAMA 2006;295:306–13.
6. Baigent C, Blackwell L, Collins R, et al, Antithrombotic Trialists' (ATT) Collaboration. Aspirin in the primary and secondary prevention of vascular disease: collaborative meta-analysis of individual participant data from randomised trials. Lancet 2009;373:1849–60.
7. Helton TJ, Bavry AA, Kumbhani DJ, et al. Incremental effect of clopidogrel on important outcomes in patients with cardiovascular disease: a meta-analysis of randomized trials. Am J Cardiovasc Drugs 2007;7:289–97.
8. Berger JS, Bhatt DL, Cannon CP, et al. The relative efficacy and safety of clopidogrel in women and men a sex-specific collaborative meta-analysis. J Am Coll Cardiol 2009;54:1935–45.
9. Bhatt DL, Fox KA, Hacke W, et al. CHARISMA Investigators. Clopidogrel and aspirin versus aspirin alone for the prevention of atherothrombotic events. N Engl J Med 2006;354:1706–17.
10. Mehta SR, Bassand JP, Chrolavicius S, et al. CURRENT-OASIS 7 Investigators, Dose comparisons of clopidogrel and aspirin in acute coronary syndromes. N Engl J Med 2010;363:930–42.
11. Wiviott SD, Braunwald E, McCabe CH, et al. TRITON-TIMI 38 Investigators. Prasugrel versus clopidogrel in patients with acute coronary syndromes. N Engl J Med 2007;357:2001–15.
12. Hochholzer W, Wiviott SD, Antman EM, et al. Predictors of bleeding and time dependence of association of bleeding with mortality: insights from the Trial to Assess Improvement in Therapeutic Outcomes by Optimizing Platelet Inhibition With

Prasugrel—Thrombolysis in Myocardial Infarction 38 (TRITON-TIMI 38). Circulation 2011;123:2681–9.

13. Wallentin L, Becker RC, Budaj A, et al. Ticagrelor versus clopidogrel in patients with acute coronary syndromes. N Engl J Med 2009;361:1045–57.

14. Barrett-Connor E. Sex differences in coronary heart disease. Why are women so superior? The 1995 Ancel Keys Lecture. Circulation 1997;95:252–64.

15. Xing D, Nozell S, Chen YF, et al. Estrogen and mechanisms of vascular protection. Arterioscler Thromb Vasc Biol 2009;29:289–95.

16. Vaidya D, Becker DM, Bittner V, et al. Ageing, menopause, and ischaemic heart disease mortality in England, Wales, and the United States: modelling study of national mortality data. BMJ 2011;343:d5170.

17. Medical Research Council. Risk of thromboembolic disease in women taking oral contraceptives. BMJ 1967;2:355–9.

18. McGregor L, Morazain R, Renaud S. Effect of different concentrations of an oral contraceptive and of pregnancy on platelet functions and platelet phospholipids fatty acid composition in rats. In: Serneri GG, Prentice CM, editors. Haemostasis and thrombosis, vol. 15. New York: Academic Press Inc; 1979. p. 565–70.

19. Uzunova A, Ramey E, Ramwell PW. Effect of testosterone, sex and age on experimentally induced arterial thrombosis. Nature 1976;261:712–3.

20. Johnson M, Ramey E, Ramwell PW. Sex and age differences in human platelet aggregation. Nature 1975;253:355–7.

21. Emms H, Lewis GP. Sex and hormonal influences on platelet sensitivity and coagulation in the rat. Br J Pharmacol 1985;86:557–63.

22. Emms H, Lewis GP. The effect of synthetic ovarian hormones on an in vivo model of thrombosis in the rat. Br J Pharmacol 1985;84:243–8.

23. Johnson M, Ramey E, Ramwell PW. Androgen-mediated sensitivity in platelet aggregation. Am J Physiol 1977;232:H381–5.

24. Leng XH, Hong SY, Larrucea S, et al. Platelets of female mice are intrinsically more sensitive to agonists than are platelets of males. Arterioscler Thromb Vasc Biol 2004;24:376–81.

25. Higashiura K, Mathur RS, Halushka PV. Gender-related differences in androgen regulation of thromboxane A2 receptors in rat aortic smooth-muscle cells. J Cardiovasc Pharmacol 1997;29:311–5.

26. Ajayi AA, Hercule H, Cory J, et al. Gender difference in vascular and platelet reactivity to thromboxane A(2)-mimetic U46619 and to endothelial dependent vasodilation in Zucker fatty (hypertensive, hyperinsulinemic) diabetic rats. Diabetes Res Clin Pract 2003;59:11–24.

27. McGill DA, Ardlie NG. Abnormal platelet reactivity in men with premature coronary heart disease. Coron Artery Dis 1994;5:889–900.

28. Kurrelmeyer K, Becker L, Becker D, et al. Platelet hyperreactivity in women from families with premature atherosclerosis. J Am Med Womens Assoc 2003;58:272–7.

29. Yee DL, Sun CW, Bergeron AL, et al. Aggregometry detects platelet hyperreactivity in healthy individuals. Blood 2005;106:2723–9.

30. Santimone I, Di Castelnuovo A, De Curtis A, et al, MOLI-SANI Project Investigators. White blood cell count, sex and age are major determinants of heterogeneity of platelet indices in an adult general population: results from the MOLI-SANI project. Haematologica 2011;96:1180–8.

31. Meade TW, Vickers MV, Thompson SG, et al. Epidemiological characteristics of platelet aggregability. Br Med J (Clin Res Ed) 1985;290:428–32.

32. Becker DM, Segal J, Vaidya D, et al. Sex differences in platelet reactivity and response to low-dose aspirin therapy. JAMA 2006;295:1420–7.

33. Faraday N, Goldschmidt-Clermont PJ, Bray PF. Gender differences in platelet GPIIb-IIIa activation. Thromb Haemost 1997;77:748–54.

34. Egan KM, Lawson JA, Fries S, et al. COX-2-derived prostacyclin confers atheroprotection on female mice. Science 2004;306:1954–7.

35. Bar J, Lahav J, Hod M, et al. Regulation of platelet aggregation and adenosine triphosphate release in vitro by 17beta-estradiol and medroxyprogesterone acetate in postmenopausal women. Thromb Haemost 2000;84:695–700.

36. Jayachandran M, Miller VM. Human platelets contain estrogen receptor alpha, caveolin-1 and estrogen receptor associated proteins. Platelets 2003;14:75–81.

37. Mendelsohn ME, Karas RH. The protective effects of estrogen on the cardiovascular system. N Engl J Med 1999;340:1801–11.

38. Harrison MJ, Weisblatt E. A sex difference in the effect of aspirin on "spontaneous" platelet aggregation in whole blood. Thromb Haemost 1983;50:773–4.

39. Spranger M, Aspey BS, Harrison MJ. Sex difference in antithrombotic effect of aspirin. Stroke 1989;20:34–7.

40. Escolar G, Bastida E, Garrido M, et al. Sex-related differences in the effects of aspirin on the interaction of platelets with subendothelium. Thromb Res 1986;44:837–47.

41. Kelton JG, Hirsh J, Carter CJ, et al. Sex differences in the antithrombotic effects of aspirin. Blood 1978;52:1073–6.

42. Qayyum R, Becker DM, Yanek LR, et al. Platelet inhibition by aspirin 81 and 325 mg/day in men versus women without clinically apparent cardiovascular disease. Am J Cardiol 2008;101:1359–63.

43. Ivandic BT, Giannitsis E, Schlick P, et al. Determination of aspirin responsiveness by use of whole blood platelet aggregometry. Clin Chem 2007;53:614–9.

44. Xie HG. Direct evidence for the higher frequency of CYP2C19 allelic heterozygotes in Chinese subjects than in white subjects. Clin Pharmacol Ther 1997; 62:691–2.

45. Ramsjo M, Aklillu E, Bohman L, et al. CYP2C19 activity comparison between Swedes and Koreans: effect of genotype, sex, oral contraceptive use, and smoking. Eur J Clin Pharmacol 2010;66:871–7.

46. Shuldiner AR, O'Connell JR, Bliden KP, et al. Association of cytochrome P450 2C19 genotype with the antiplatelet effect and clinical efficacy of clopidogrel therapy. JAMA 2009;302:849–57.

47. Gurbel PA, Bliden KP, Cohen E, et al. Race and sex differences in thrombogenicity: risk of ischemic events following coronary stenting. Blood Coagul Fibrinolysis 2008;19:268–75.

# Cardiogenic Shock in Women

Vijay Kunadian, MBBS, MD, MRCP[a,b,*],
Louise Coats, MRCP, PhD[b], Annapoorna S. Kini, MD, MRCP[c],
Roxana Mehran, MD[c]

**KEYWORDS**
- Cardiogenic shock • Women • Myocardial infarction
- Left ventricular assist device

Cardiogenic shock (CS) describes the physiologic state in which reduced cardiac output (CO) and resultant tissue hypoxia occur in the presence of adequate intravascular volume. Hemodynamically, this is defined as a decrease in systolic blood pressure to less than 90 mm Hg sustained for at least 30 minutes in the absence of hypovolemia, with a cardiac index less than $1.8 \ L/min/m^2$ without support or 2.0 to $2.2 \ L/min/m^2$ with support, in the presence of an increased pulmonary capillary wedge pressure (>15 mm Hg).[1,2] The clinical manifestations of CS include cool extremities, decreased urine output, and altered mental status. Cardiac power, a product of mean arterial pressure and CO, is the strongest hemodynamic correlate of outcome for patients with CS. Increasing age and female gender are independently associated with lower cardiac power.[3]

It has repeatedly been shown that women hospitalized with myocardial infarction (MI) are more likely to die than men; much of this can be attributed to their different risk profile (older age, more hypertension, hypercholesterolemia, diabetes mellitus, and congestive heart failure).[4–7] There is a higher prevalence of CS among women, which raises important issues regarding targeting treatment.[8–10]

This article examines the prevalence, cause, pathophysiology, and therapeutic options for CS among women. The key points are summarized in **Box 1**.

## THE SCOPE OF THE PROBLEM

Despite substantial improvement in mortality from cardiovascular disease, mainly due to the success of primary and secondary prevention strategies, it remains the leading cause of death among women in the developed world.[11] Both in-hospital (women 11.9% vs men 6.9%, $P<.0001$) and 12-month (women 22% vs men 14.1%, $P<.0001$) mortality following MI are significantly higher in women and influenced by age, diabetes, pulmonary edema, CS, cardiac arrest, infarct site, and likelihood of undergoing primary percutaneous coronary intervention (PPCI).[12] Mortality is now increasing in younger women in line with increasing levels of obesity in the population.[13]

Among those patients hospitalized with MI, CS is the foremost cause of death, complicating up to 10% of admissions.[9,10,14–17] Women experience CS more often than men (11.6% vs 8.3%, $P = .01$) in the setting of ST elevation MI and, notably, the prevalence is greater among young women (aged 30–59 years, odds ratio [OR] 1.76).[10,17]

### In-Hospital Mortality due to Cardiogenic Shock

The introduction of early revascularization strategies and mechanical ventricular support has seen short-term mortality caused by CS decrease from 70% to 80% in the 1970s to around 50% to 60% in the 1990s.[1,14,15,18] However, registry

Disclosures: None of the authors have any conflict of interest to disclose.
[a] Institute of Cellular Medicine, Faculty of Medical Sciences, Newcastle University, Newcastle upon Tyne, UK
[b] Cardiothoracic Centre, Freeman Hospital, Newcastle upon Tyne Hospitals, NHS Foundation Trust, Newcastle upon Tyne, UK
[c] Mount Sinai School of Medicine, One Gustave L. Levy Place, New York, NY 10029, USA
* Corresponding author. Institute of Cellular Medicine, Faculty of Medical Sciences, Newcastle University, 3rd Floor William Leech Building, Newcastle upon Tyne, NE2 4HH, UK.
E-mail address: vijay.kunadian@ncl.ac.uk

Intervent Cardiol Clin 1 (2012) 231–243
doi:10.1016/j.iccl.2012.01.006
2211-7458/12/$ – see front matter © 2012 Elsevier Inc. All rights reserved.

**Box 1**
**Key points**

- CS is the leading cause of death following MI and complicates up to 10% of cases
- Women have higher in-hospital mortality than men following acute MI
- There is increased prevalence of CS among women
- Special conditions, such as spontaneous coronary artery dissection, peripartum cardiomyopathy, coronary artery spasm, and takotsubo cardiomyopathy, lead to cardiogenic shock, particularly among women

studies evaluating the impact of CS on in-hospital mortality among women compared with men have shown varied outcomes.[8,19–21] Edep and Brown[8] showed that, after multivariate adjustment, women were at increased risk of in-hospital mortality (OR 1.4, $P = .01$) compared with men in the setting of CS following acute MI. However, in the SHOCK (Should we Emergently Revascularize Occluded Coronaries for Cardiogenic Shock) registry, after adjustment for differences in patient demographics and treatment approaches, there was no significant difference in in-hospital mortality (women 63.4% vs men 59.3%, OR 1.16, 95% confidence interval [CI] 0.87–1.55, $P = .252$) among patients presenting with CS in the setting of acute MI.[20] In the ALKK (Arbeitsgemeinschaft Leitende Kardiologische Krankenhausärzte) registry, female gender was not a predictor of in-hospital mortality in patients with CS (OR 0.9, 95% CI 0.5–1.5).[21] These studies were performed at different time intervals using different treatment strategies, which might explain the differences in in-hospital outcomes, particularly among women.

## CAUSES OF CARDIOGENIC SHOCK

Most cases of CS occur in the context of MI, with left ventricular failure being the primary mechanism. Mechanical ischemic conditions such as acute severe mitral regurgitation, ventricular septal rupture, and right ventricular infarction account for most of the remainder.[22] Women are more likely to have mechanical complications such as ventricular septal or papillary muscle rupture (women 7.7% vs men 3.5%, $P = .003$) and severe mitral regurgitation (women 11.4% vs men 7.1%, $P = .014$).[20,22] Understanding the relationship of gender to cause may provide insights into the pathophysiology. The causes of CS and the presence of a gender

preference under various conditions are presented in **Table 1**.

## RISK FACTORS FOR DEVELOPMENT OF CARDIOGENIC SHOCK

During the thrombolytic era, women presenting with MI were, on average, 10 years older than men, with a greater prevalence of type 1 and 2 diabetes mellitus, hypertension, peripheral vascular disease, preceding cerebrovascular events, and symptomatic congestive heart failure, as shown in **Table 2**.[10,16,17] Women fared worse than men following acute MI, with increased mortality and, in particular, diabetic women were at high risk for in-hospital and 1-year mortality.[23] In the context of patients receiving thrombolysis for acute ST elevation MI, age, systolic blood pressure, heart rate, and Killip class on presentation have been identified as independent risk factors for development of CS.[24]

## PATHOPHYSIOLOGY

The mechanism of shock is best considered in terms of left ventricular ischemia. Autopsy studies suggest that, in the absence of tachyarrhythmia, a loss of more than 40% of myocardium is necessary to develop CS.[25] Shock can be discussed at the level of the occluded coronary artery, the damaged microvasculature, the myocyte, and the hormonal/endocrine response.

In ST segment elevation MI, no gender difference has been shown in terms of the extent of coronary artery disease, the presence of left main stem lesions, or the site of infarct.[16,26] However, men have often had prior ischemic insults and the presence of a collateral circulation may offer a survival benefit if CS occurs.[27]

### Microvascular Dysfunction

Myocardial ischemia in the presence of nonobstructive coronary arteries is more commonly seen in women.[28] The theory that this is caused by endothelial and/or microvascular disease is supported by findings of abnormal coronary blood flow response to vasoactive stimuli, increased transmyocardial lipoperoxide activity, and abnormal myocardial phosphorus metabolism.[29–31] This condition is associated with a reduced coronary flow reserve.[32]

Recent work suggests that plaque rupture and ulceration are common findings in MI and nonobstructive coronary arteries, a condition that is also more common in women (**Fig. 1**). In addition, late gadolinium enhancement on magnetic resonance imaging is common in this cohort of women,

**Table 1**
**Causes of cardiogenic shock**

| Condition | Gender Predilection | References |
|---|---|---|
| **Acute myocardial infarction** | | |
|   Primary ventricular dysfunction | | |
|     Loss of >40% of left ventricular mass | | |
|     Loss of <40% of left ventricular myocardial with arrhythmia | | |
|   Mechanical defects | | |
|     Septal, papillary muscle, chordal, or free wall rupture | More common in women | 22,91–93 |
|     Right ventricular infarction | No difference | 94 |
| **Cardiomyopathy** | | |
|   Dilated | No difference | |
|   Hypertrophic | No difference | |
|   Peripartum | Exclusively affects women | |
|   Takotsubo | Predominantly affects women (>90%) | 95 |
|   Tachycardia induced | | |
| **Valvular heart disease** | | |
|   Aortic stenosis or regurgitation | | |
|   Mitral stenosis or regurgitation | | |
| **Miscellaneous** | | |
|   Infective endocarditis | | |
|   Aortic dissection | | |
|   Myocardial contusion/valve trauma | | |
|   Valvular obstruction by thrombus, vegetation, or tumor | | |
|   Prosthetic valve dysfunction | | |
|   Pericardial disease | | |
|   Cardiac tamponade | | |
|   Severe myocarditis | | |
|   Prolonged cardiopulmonary bypass | | |
|   Postcardiotomy shock | | |
|   Iatrogenic | | |

**Table 2**
**Risk profile associated with coronary artery disease and cardiogenic shock**

| Risk Profile | Gender | References |
|---|---|---|
| Type 1 diabetes mellitus | Women | 10,16,64 |
| Type 2 diabetes mellitus | Women | 10,16,64 |
| Hypertension | Women | 10,64 |
| Peripheral vascular disease | Women | 10 |
| Previous cerebrovascular events | Women | 10 |
| Smoking | Men | 10 |
| Previous infarct | Men | 10 |
| Previous revascularization | Men | 10 |
| Previous and current congestive cardiac failure | Women | 10,64 |

with an ischemic pattern of injury being most evident. Vasospasm and embolism are possible mechanisms of ischemic injury without plaque disruption.[33] Vasospasm causing infarction may reflect severe endothelial dysfunction linking the pathophysiology of these 2 clinical pictures. The assumption therefore must be that female susceptibility to endothelial dysfunction and microvascular disease also coexists with obstructive coronary artery disease and may provide one explanation for why women are seemingly at higher risk of CS.

Women with acute coronary syndromes have similar or better left ventricular ejection fractions and fewer high-risk lesions than men, despite more frequent heart failure symptoms. In the context of higher levels of hypertension, a component of diastolic dysfunction must be assumed.[10,26] Gender differences in myocardial response to injury at a cellular level and cardiac

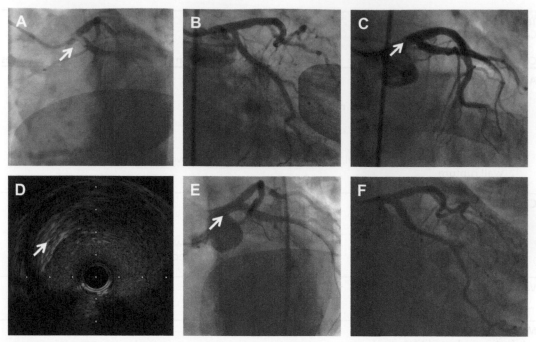

**Fig. 1.** Case example of a 59 year old woman who presented with CS in the setting of STEMI (late presentation with ongoing symptoms). Initial angio showed thrombus in left main stem (LMS), and circumflex artery (A, arrow). Export aspiration cleared the thrombus (B) with evidence of haziness in the ostial LMS (C) confirmed on intravascular ultrasound (IVUS) as a plaque in ostial LMS (D) which was treated successfully with LMS stenting (E), with widely patent stent at 3-month follow-up angio (F).

remodeling have been observed, with women exhibiting reduced hypertrophy after infarction compared with men.[34]

### Protective Effects of Estrogen

The later onset of ischemic heart disease in women reflects the pivotal effect of menopause. Animal studies have shown female gender to be protective against ischemia reperfusion injury, supporting other evidence that estrogen offers a protective effect in coronary artery disease.[35–37] This in part explains why women manifest symptoms and present later than men. However, diabetes mellitus negates the protective effect of estrogen and is a stronger prognostic factor after MI in women compared with men.[37]

Furthermore, the systemic inflammatory response syndrome (SIRS), which can occur during CS, leads to vasodilatation and impaired perfusion of the intestines, resulting in transmigration of bacteria and sepsis. Increased levels of cytokine, tumor necrosis factor (TNF) α, interleukin-6 (IL-6), complement, procalcitonin, neopterin, and C-reactive protein are identified in SIRS. IL-6 and TNF α have myocardial depressant effects, with the latter inducing endothelial dysfunction.[38–40] Women tend to have less inflammation through the protective effect of estrogen.

### Excess Bleeding

Women are at higher risk of bleeding, in part because of their more advanced age and other comorbidities. Additional anticoagulation is necessary for the use of left ventricular assist devices (LVADs) in the setting of CS. However, bleeding and blood transfusion in the context of CS complicating MI may contribute to increased mortality.[41]

## CARDIOGENIC SHOCK IN SPECIAL SITUATIONS
### Peripartum Cardiomyopathy

Development of acute heart failure in the late stages of pregnancy and several months beyond childbirth is termed peripartum cardiomyopathy and occurs in around 1:3000 to 1:4000 live births. Development of CS in this setting has previously been described and administration of the prolactin inhibitor bromocriptine has been suggested as specific therapy.[42] Evidence suggests that a derivate of the hormone prolactin, which is upregulated in the postpartum period, mediates cardiomyopathy by initiating cell apoptosis and disruption of capillaries, which then leads to heart failure and myocardial damage.[43,44]

## Spontaneous Coronary Artery Dissection

Spontaneous coronary artery dissection (SCAD), most commonly observed among women, can present with cardiac arrest and CS requiring an LVAD.[45,46] SCAD is a rare condition that typically affects young to middle-aged women, especially during the peripartum or early postpartum period. Although hypertension, collagen disorders, intense physical effort, and blunt chest trauma have been considered to be predisposing factors, the cause and pathogenesis of SCAD are unclear. SCAD presents frequently with sudden cardiac death or acute coronary syndrome and can also present with left ventricular failure, CS, and cardiac tamponade. Coronary angiography, revascularization with adjunctive mechanical support, and even cardiac transplant have been used in its management.[47]

## Takotsubo Cardiomyopathy

CS has been reported in the setting of takotsubo cardiomyopathy (TTC), a condition predominantly affecting women, specifically in association with anorexia nervosa and pheochromocytoma.[48,49] TTC, also known as transient left ventricular ballooning syndrome or stress-induced cardiomyopathy, is characterized by transient left ventricular dysfunction in the absence of significant angiographic coronary stenoses, provoked by an episode of emotional or physical stress. Recovery is excellent in most cases when appropriate treatment is instigated early.[50] Among those presenting with CS, there is greater prevalence of heart failure symptoms, an apical ballooning pattern, significant mitral regurgitation, and increased cardiac biomarker levels. Several treatment strategies, including levosimendan, dobutamine, and extracorporeal membrane exchange, have been used in the treatment of CS complicating TTC.[51–53]

## Coronary Artery Spasm

There are case reports of women experiencing CS in the setting of severe coronary artery spasm,[54–56] particularly in women with asthma[54] and hyperthyroidism.[57] The management of this condition requires intracoronary vasodilators, such as nitrates, and, in the setting of severe hypotension, inotropes, and intra-aortic balloon pumps (IABPs) may be beneficial.

## THERAPEUTIC OPTIONS

Various therapeutic strategies have been used in the management of patients with CS and are discussed in the following paragraphs. However, studies evaluating therapies specifically targeting women are lacking.

## Inotropes: Dopamine Versus Norepinephrine

In the setting of CS, inotropes help maintain blood pressure and organ perfusion. In a multicenter, randomized trial, patients with shock (44% of which were female patients) were assigned to receive either dopamine or norepinephrine as first-line vasopressor therapy to restore and maintain blood pressure. Although there was no significant difference in the rate of death between patients with shock who were treated with dopamine as the first-line vasopressor agent and those who were treated with norepinephrine, the use of dopamine was associated with a greater number of adverse events, which consisted mainly of arrhythmias.[58]

## Levosimendan

Levosimendan is a new calcium sensitizer and K-ATP channel opener that improves myocardial contractility. In patients with severe and refractory CS complicating acute MI, levosimendan added to current therapy can lead to early and sustained hemodynamic improvement and, compared with enoximone, a phosphodiesterase III inhibitor, may contribute to improved survival. Furthermore, short-term hemodynamic effects compare favorably with those seen after invasive IABP placement.[59,60]

## Adjunctive Pharmacotherapy

### Antiplatelet agents
Given that acute MI is the commonest cause of CS, antiplatelet therapy plays an important role in the management of these patients. In a nonrandomized study, the use bivalirudin with provisional GP IIb/IIIa has been favorable during PPCI in the setting of CS.[61] Abciximab has been used in the setting of CS with a high procedure success rate with improved outcomes.[62] However, both in the era of thrombolysis and more recently in the setting of PPCI, it has been shown that women are less likely to receive aspirin on admission and glycoprotein IIb/IIIa inhibitors.[10,16,63,64]

### Nitric oxide synthase inhibitors
Nitric oxide (NO) is a potent vasodilator exhibiting positive inotropic effects at low levels and negative inotropic effects at high levels. Release of inflammatory cytokines that trigger NO overproduction in the heart and blood vessels are associated with large MI. It is possible that NO synthase inhibitors reduce the direct deleterious

effect of NO on the myocardium and induce vaso-constriction, thus improving mean arterial pressure and coronary perfusion pressure, and may be efficacious in the treatment of CS. Although a small randomized trial suggested some benefit with NO synthase inhibitors,[65] a further study using tilarginine, an isoform nonselective NO synthase inhibitor (1-mg/kg bolus and 5-h infusion), did not reduce mortality among patients with refractory CS complicating MI despite an open infarct artery (in this study, only 26% of patients were women).[2]

## Reperfusion and Revascularization Strategies

### Thrombolysis

Historically, perhaps in light of higher rates of contraindications among women, thrombolysis has been underused and door-to-needle times in those treated have been longer than for men.[66,67] Despite this, rates of reperfusion between the genders have been comparable.[68] Thrombolysis has been unable to reduce the mortality gap seen between the genders.[69] Although there are no studies specifically targeting women, for patients with CS following ST elevation MI presenting to centers with a thrombolysis facility only, a strategy of early thrombolysis and IABP followed by immediate transfer for revascularization should be considered.[70]

### PPCI

PPCI is now well established as the preferred treatment strategy for ST elevation MI.[71] Despite similar rates of PPCI being shown in women, in terms of number of vessels treated and use of drug-eluting versus bare metal stents, there is a lower success rate (94.7% vs 95.9%, $P = .002$) and higher in-hospital mortality (9.8% vs 4.3%) even after adjustment for risk factors.[16] The SHOCK trial found significant mortality reduction with early revascularization,[72] and no gender difference in early outcome has been observed in this subset with CS.[19] Although current guidelines recommend multivessel percutaneous coronary intervention (PCI) in the setting of CS, there are no randomized trials comparing culprit vessel versus multivessel PCI in the setting of CS complicating ST elevation MI.

### Intracoronary Pharmacotherapy

Intracoronary pharmacotherapy such as intracoronary abciximab has been shown to improve coronary artery blood flow, myocardial perfusion, myocardial salvage, left ventricular function, and mortality.[73-76] Abciximab attenuates endothelial dysfunction after coronary stenting and

demonstrates antiinflammatory properties by inhibiting smooth muscle cell migration and proliferation.[77] Data from the American College of Cardiology/National Cardiovascular Data Registry showed that no glycoprotein inhibitor use during PCI was a predictor of death among patients with acute MI presenting with CS and undergoing emergency percutaneous coronary intervention.[78]

In clinical studies, intracoronary adenosine has been shown to improve outcomes, coronary flow, and corrected Thrombolysis in Myocardial Infarction (TIMI) frame count.[76,79,80] However, no significant benefit has been seen in the setting of PPCI in terms of improving perfusion.[81] Although randomized studies using intracoronary pharmacotherapy are lacking in the CS setting, adenosine in combination with IABP, and glycoprotein IIb/IIIa inhibitor have been used favorably in the management of profound CS.[82]

### LVADs

Although several LVADs have been studied in CS, the benefit of these devices specifically among women has not been evaluated. A brief overview of these devices and their use in CS is given here.

### IABP

In the thrombolytic therapy era, treatment of patients with CS caused by left ventricular failure, IABP (Maquet Inc., Wayne, NJ), and revascularization by balloon angioplasty or coronary artery bypass surgery was associated with lower in-hospital mortality than standard medical therapy.[70] Recently, randomized trials have shown no benefit with routine IABP insertion among patients with severe left ventricular dysfunction and extensive coronary disease,[83] and among patients with acute anterior MI in the absence of shock.[84] Furthermore, a meta-analysis did not support IABP therapy adjunctive to PPCI in the setting of CS.[85] All available observational data concerning IABP therapy in the setting of CS is hampered by bias and confounding. With contemporary treatment strategies including PPCI and more potent pharmacotherapy, whether IABP would be of benefit in the setting of CS is currently being evaluated (**Fig. 2**).[86]

### Impella and TandemHeart

In patients presenting with CS caused by acute MI, the use of a percutaneously placed Impella LP 2.5 (Abiomed Danvers, MA; **Fig. 3**, **Table 3**), an LVAD, is feasible and safe, and provides superior hemodynamic support compared with

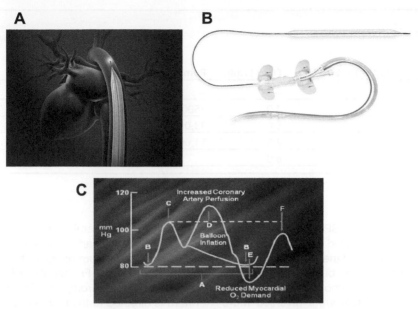

**Fig. 2.** IABP. (*A*) SENSATION PLUS 8-Fr-50-mL intra-aortic balloon (IAB) catheter in the aorta. (*B*) SENSATION PLUS 8-Fr 50-mL IAB catheter with STATLOCK IAB stabilization devices. (*C*) Timing assessment: A, 1 cardiac cycle; B, unassisted end diastole; C, unassisted systole; D, augmented diastole; E, assisted end diastole; F, assisted systole. (*Courtesy of* Maquet, UK; with permission.)

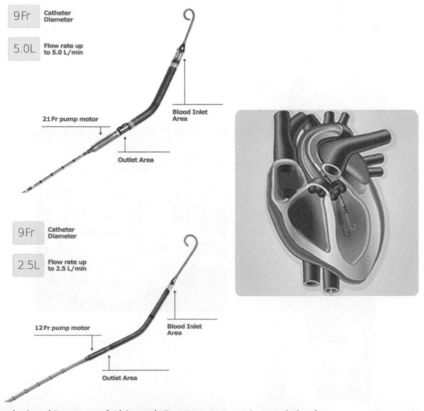

**Fig. 3.** Impella device. (*Courtesy of* Abiomed, Danvers, MA; with permission.)

**Table 3**
**Comparison of different LVADs**

| LVAD | Catheter Size (Fr) | Flow L/min | Pump Speed (rpm) | Duration of Use | Site of Insertion |
|---|---|---|---|---|---|
| IABP | 7–8 | — | — | 48–72 h[a] | FA |
| TandemHeart | — | 4.0 | 7500 | 14 d | FA |
| Impella 5.0 | 9 | 5.0 | 33,000 | 10 d | FA |
| Impella 2.5 | 9 | 2.5 | 51,000 | 10 d | FA |
| AB5000 | 32–42 | 6.0 | — | >25 d | TC |

*Abbreviations:* FA, femoral artery; TC, transcardiac.
   [a] For a single catheter.

standard treatment using IABP.[87] A meta-analysis that consisted of controlled trials to evaluate potential benefits of percutaneous LVADs did not result in improved mortality but did help improve hemodynamics.[88] Furthermore, hemodynamic and metabolic parameters were reversed more effectively by the TandemHeart ventricular assist device (VAD) (CardiacAssist, Pittsburgh, PA) than by standard treatment with IABP, albeit with increased bleeding and limb ischemia using TandemHeart (**Fig. 4**, see **Table 3**).[89]

## AB5000 VAD

AB5000 VAD (Abiomed, Danvers, MA) provides paracorporeal, univentricular, or biventricular pulsatile hemodynamic support (**Fig. 5**, see **Table 3**). Left heart cannulation is achieved through the left atrium or apex of the left ventricle using a 32-Fr or 42-Fr cannula; right heart cannulation is achieved through the right atrium. Arterial return is directed to the pulmonary artery or aorta using a 10-mm graft. The AB5000 ventricle is driven by a pneumatic console that allows for patient ambulation and delivers up to 6 L of blood per minute. A voluntary US registry study (consisting of 32% female patients) showed that the AB5000 VAD can restore normal hemodynamics and support recovery of native cardiac function in most survivors when conventional therapies fail in CS following MI. In this study, the VAD was in place for an average of 25 days

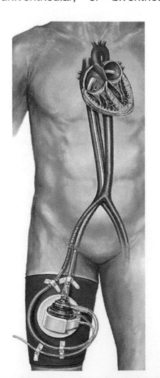

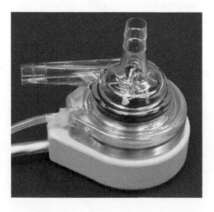

**Fig. 4.** TandemHeart. (*Courtesy of* CardiacAssist, Pittsburgh, PA, USA; with permission.)

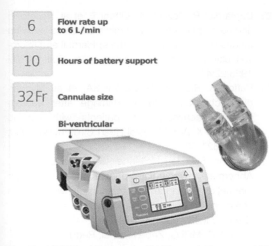

| 6 | Flow rate up to 6 L/min |
| 10 | Hours of battery support |
| 32Fr | Cannulae size |

Bi-ventricular

**Fig. 5.** AB5000. (*Courtesy of* Abiomed, Danvers, MA; with permission.)

before a satisfactory native cardiac function was achieved.[90]

## SUMMARY

CS is the leading cause of death, complicating up to 10% of admissions among patients presenting with MI. There is increased prevalence of CS among women. Special conditions such as SCAD, peripartum cardiomyopathy, takotsubo cardiomyopathy, and coronary artery spasm lead to CS, particularly among women. Although women have increased prevalence of CS, they are underrepresented in clinical studies. Randomized clinical trials investigating optimal strategies to improve outcomes among patients with CS not only among women but also among the entire cohort are currently lacking and warrant further investigation.

## REFERENCES

1. Hochman JS, Sleeper LA, Webb JG, et al. Early revascularization in acute myocardial infarction complicated by cardiogenic shock. N Engl J Med 1999;341:625–34.
2. Alexander JH, Reynolds HR, Stebbins AL, et al. Effect of tilarginine acetate in patients with acute myocardial infarction and cardiogenic shock: the TRIUMPH randomized controlled trial. JAMA 2007; 297:1657–66.
3. Fincke R, Hochman JS, Lowe AM, et al. Cardiac power is the strongest hemodynamic correlate of mortality in cardiogenic shock: a report from the SHOCK trial registry. J Am Coll Cardiol 2004;44:340–8.
4. Kober L, Torp-Pedersen C, Ottesen M, et al. Influence of gender on short- and long-term mortality after acute myocardial infarction. TRACE study group. Am J Cardiol 1996;77:1052–6.
5. Coronado BE, Griffith JL, Beshansky JR, et al. Hospital mortality in women and men with acute cardiac ischemia: a prospective multicenter study. J Am Coll Cardiol 1997;29:1490–6.
6. Robinson K, Conroy RM, Mulcahy R, et al. Risk factors and in-hospital course of first episode of myocardial infarction or acute coronary insufficiency in women. J Am Coll Cardiol 1988;11:932–6.
7. Malacrida R, Genoni M, Maggioni AP, et al. A comparison of the early outcome of acute myocardial infarction in women and men. The Third International Study of Infarct Survival Collaborative Group. N Engl J Med 1998;338:8–14.
8. Edep ME, Brown DL. Effect of early revascularization on mortality from cardiogenic shock complicating acute myocardial infarction in California. Am J Cardiol 2000;85:1185–8.
9. Goldberg RJ, Gore JM, Alpert JS, et al. Cardiogenic shock after acute myocardial infarction. Incidence and mortality from a community-wide perspective, 1975 to 1988. N Engl J Med 1991;325:1117–22.
10. Akhter N, Milford-Beland S, Roe MT, et al. Gender differences among patients with acute coronary syndromes undergoing percutaneous coronary intervention in the American College of Cardiology-National Cardiovascular Data Registry (ACC-NCDR). Am Heart J 2009;157:141–8.
11. Gholizadeh L, Davidson P. More similarities than differences: an international comparison of CVD mortality and risk factors in women. Health Care Women Int 2008;29:3–22.
12. Sadowski M, Gasior M, Gierlotka M, et al. Gender-related differences in mortality after ST-segment elevation myocardial infarction: a large multicentre national registry. EuroIntervention 2011;6:1068–72.
13. Ford ES, Ajani UA, Croft JB, et al. Explaining the decrease in U.S. deaths from coronary disease, 1980-2000. N Engl J Med 2007;356:2388–98.
14. Babaev A, Frederick PD, Pasta DJ, et al. Trends in management and outcomes of patients with acute myocardial infarction complicated by cardiogenic shock. JAMA 2005;294:448–54.
15. Goldberg RJ, Samad NA, Yarzebski J, et al. Temporal trends in cardiogenic shock complicating acute myocardial infarction. N Engl J Med 1999; 340:1162–8.
16. Benamer H, Tafflet M, Bataille S, et al. Female gender is an independent predictor of in-hospital mortality after STEMI in the era of primary PCI: insights from the greater Paris area PCI Registry. EuroIntervention 2011;6:1073–9.
17. Vaccarino V, Parsons L, Every NR, et al. Sex-based differences in early mortality after myocardial infarction. National Registry of Myocardial Infarction 2 Participants. N Engl J Med 1999;341:217–25.

18. Hochman JS, Sleeper LA, Godfrey E, et al. SHould we emergently revascularize Occluded Coronaries for cardiogenic shocK: an international randomized trial of emergency PTCA/CABG-trial design. The SHOCK Trial Study Group. Am Heart J 1999;137: 313–21.

19. Antoniucci D, Migliorini A, Moschi G, et al. Does gender affect the clinical outcome of patients with acute myocardial infarction complicated by cardiogenic shock who undergo percutaneous coronary intervention? Catheter Cardiovasc Interv 2003;59: 423–8.

20. Wong SC, Sleeper LA, Monrad ES, et al. Absence of gender differences in clinical outcomes in patients with cardiogenic shock complicating acute myocardial infarction. A report from the SHOCK Trial Registry. J Am Coll Cardiol 2001;38:1395–401.

21. Zeymer U, Vogt A, Zahn R, et al. Predictors of in-hospital mortality in 1333 patients with acute myocardial infarction complicated by cardiogenic shock treated with primary percutaneous coronary intervention (PCI); results of the primary PCI registry of the Arbeitsgemeinschaft Leitende Kardiologische Krankenhausarzte (ALKK). Eur Heart J 2004;25: 322–8.

22. Hochman JS, Boland J, Sleeper LA, et al. Current spectrum of cardiogenic shock and effect of early revascularization on mortality. Results of an International Registry. SHOCK Registry Investigators. Circulation 1995;91:873–81.

23. Greenland P, Reicher-Reiss H, Goldbourt U, et al. In-hospital and 1-year mortality in 1,524 women after myocardial infarction. Comparison with 4,315 men. Circulation 1991;83:484–91.

24. Hasdai D, Califf RM, Thompson TD, et al. Predictors of cardiogenic shock after thrombolytic therapy for acute myocardial infarction. J Am Coll Cardiol 2000;35:136–43.

25. Alonso DR, Scheidt S, Post M, et al. Pathophysiology of cardiogenic shock. Quantification of myocardial necrosis, clinical, pathologic and electrocardiographic correlations. Circulation 1973;48:588–96.

26. Fabijanic D, Culic V, Bozic I, et al. Gender differences in in-hospital mortality and mechanisms of death after the first acute myocardial infarction. Ann Saudi Med 2006;26:455–60.

27. Antoniucci D, Valenti R, Moschi G, et al. Relation between preintervention angiographic evidence of coronary collateral circulation and clinical and angiographic outcomes after primary angioplasty or stenting for acute myocardial infarction. Am J Cardiol 2002;89:121–5.

28. Diver DJ, Bier JD, Ferreira PE, et al. Clinical and arteriographic characterization of patients with unstable angina without critical coronary arterial narrowing (from the TIMI-IIIA Trial). Am J Cardiol 1994; 74:531–7.

29. Bugiardini R, Pozzati A, Ottani F, et al. Vasotonic angina: a spectrum of ischemic syndromes involving functional abnormalities of the epicardial and microvascular coronary circulation. J Am Coll Cardiol 1993;22:417–25.

30. Buffon A, Rigattieri S, Santini SA, et al. Myocardial ischemia-reperfusion damage after pacing-induced tachycardia in patients with cardiac syndrome X. Am J Physiol Heart Circ Physiol 2000; 279:H2627–33.

31. Buchthal SD, den Hollander JA, Merz CN, et al. Abnormal myocardial phosphorus-31 nuclear magnetic resonance spectroscopy in women with chest pain but normal coronary angiograms. N Engl J Med 2000;342:829–35.

32. Opherk D, Mall G, Zebe H, et al. Reduction of coronary reserve: a mechanism for angina pectoris in patients with arterial hypertension and normal coronary arteries. Circulation 1984;69:1–7.

33. Reynolds HR, Srichai MB, Iqbal SN, et al. Mechanisms of myocardial infarction in women without angiographically obstructive coronary artery disease. Circulation 2011;124:1414–25.

34. Crabbe DL, Dipla K, Ambati S, et al. Gender differences in post-infarction hypertrophy in end-stage failing hearts. J Am Coll Cardiol 2003;41:300–6.

35. Barrett-Connor E, Bush TL. Estrogen and coronary heart disease in women. JAMA 1991;265:1861–7.

36. Ostadal B, Netuka I, Maly J, et al. Gender differences in cardiac ischemic injury and protection–experimental aspects. Exp Biol Med (Maywood) 2009;234:1011–9.

37. Sowers JR. Diabetes mellitus and cardiovascular disease in women. Arch Intern Med 1998;158: 617–21.

38. Brunkhorst FM, Clark AL, Forycki ZF, et al. Pyrexia, procalcitonin, immune activation and survival in cardiogenic shock: the potential importance of bacterial translocation. Int J Cardiol 1999;72:3–10.

39. Theroux P, Armstrong PW, Mahaffey KW, et al. Prognostic significance of blood markers of inflammation in patients with ST-segment elevation myocardial infarction undergoing primary angioplasty and effects of pexelizumab, a C5 inhibitor: a substudy of the COMMA trial. Eur Heart J 2005;26:1964–70.

40. Debrunner M, Schuiki E, Minder E, et al. Proinflammatory cytokines in acute myocardial infarction with and without cardiogenic shock. Clin Res Cardiol 2008;97:298–305.

41. Kunadian V, Zorkun C, Gibson WJ, et al. Transfusion associated microchimerism: a heretofore little-recognized complication following transfusion. J Thromb Thrombolysis 2009;27:57–67.

42. Emmert MY, Pretre R, Ruschitzka F, et al. Peripartum cardiomyopathy with cardiogenic shock: recovery after prolactin inhibition and mechanical support. Ann Thorac Surg 2011;91:274–6.

43. Hilfiker-Kleiner D, Kaminski K, Podewski E, et al. A cathepsin D-cleaved 16 kDa form of prolactin mediates postpartum cardiomyopathy. Cell 2007; 128:589–600.

44. Hilfiker-Kleiner D, Sliwa K, Drexler H. Peripartum cardiomyopathy: recent insights in its pathophysiology. Trends Cardiovasc Med 2008;18:173–9.

45. Jacob JC, Kiernan FJ, Patel N, et al. SCAD: a rare case of cardiac arrest in a young female. Conn Med 2011;75:147–52.

46. Bergen E, Huffer L, Peele M. Survival after spontaneous coronary artery dissection presenting with ventricular fibrillation arrest. J Invasive Cardiol 2005;17:E4–6.

47. Ferrari E, Tozzi P, von Segesser LK. Spontaneous coronary artery dissection in a young woman: from emergency coronary artery bypass grafting to heart transplantation. Eur J Cardiothorac Surg 2005;28: 349–51.

48. Volman MN, Ten Kate RW, Tukkie R. Tako Tsubo cardiomyopathy, presenting with cardiogenic shock in a 24-year-old patient with anorexia nervosa. Neth J Med 2011;69:129–31.

49. Lassnig E, Weber T, Auer J, et al. Pheochromocytoma crisis presenting with shock and takotsubo-like cardiomyopathy. Int J Cardiol 2009; 134:e138–40.

50. Song BG, Park SJ, Noh HJ, et al. Clinical characteristics, and laboratory and echocardiographic findings in takotsubo cardiomyopathy presenting as cardiogenic shock. J Crit Care 2010;25:329–35.

51. De Santis V, Vitale D, Tritapepe L, et al. Use of levosimendan for cardiogenic shock in a patient with the apical ballooning syndrome. Ann Intern Med 2008; 149:365–7.

52. Abe Y, Tamura A, Kadota J. Prolonged cardiogenic shock caused by a high-dose intravenous administration of dopamine in a patient with takotsubo cardiomyopathy. Int J Cardiol 2010;141:e1–3.

53. Zegdi R, Parisot C, Sleilaty G, et al. Pheochromocytoma-induced inverted takotsubo cardiomyopathy: a case of patient resuscitation with extracorporeal life support. J Thorac Cardiovasc Surg 2008;135: 434–5.

54. Tacoy G, Kocaman SA, Balcioglu S, et al. Coronary vasospastic crisis leading to cardiogenic shock and recurrent ventricular fibrillation in a patient with long-standing asthma. J Cardiol 2008;52:300–4.

55. Lilli A, Vecchio S, Vittori G, et al. Severe diffuse coronary artery spasm in the early phase of cardiogenic shock. Int J Cardiol 2009;134:e103–4.

56. Wong A, Cheng A, Chan C, et al. Cardiogenic shock caused by severe coronary artery spasm immediately after coronary stenting. Tex Heart Inst J 2005; 32:78–80.

57. Lassnig E, Berent R, Auer J, et al. Cardiogenic shock due to myocardial infarction caused by coronary vasospasm associated with hyperthyroidism. Int J Cardiol 2003;90:333–5.

58. De Backer D, Biston P, Devriendt J, et al. Comparison of dopamine and norepinephrine in the treatment of shock. N Engl J Med 2010;362:779–89.

59. Fuhrmann JT, Schmeisser A, Schulze MR, et al. Levosimendan is superior to enoximone in refractory cardiogenic shock complicating acute myocardial infarction. Crit Care Med 2008;36:2257–66.

60. Christoph A, Prondzinsky R, Russ M, et al. Early and sustained haemodynamic improvement with levosimendan compared to intraaortic balloon counterpulsation (IABP) in cardiogenic shock complicating acute myocardial infarction. Acute Card Care 2008;10:49–57.

61. Bonello L, De Labriolle A, Roy P, et al. Bivalirudin with provisional glycoprotein IIb/IIIa inhibitors in patients undergoing primary angioplasty in the setting of cardiogenic shock. Am J Cardiol 2008; 102:287–91.

62. Zeymer U, Tebbe U, Weber M, et al. Prospective evaluation of early abciximab and primary percutaneous intervention for patients with ST elevation myocardial infarction complicated by cardiogenic shock: results of the REO-SHOCK trial. J Invasive Cardiol 2003;15:385–9.

63. Barakat K, Wilkinson P, Suliman A, et al. Acute myocardial infarction in women: contribution of treatment variables to adverse outcome. Am Heart J 2000;140:740–6.

64. Blomkalns AL, Chen AY, Hochman JS, et al. Gender disparities in the diagnosis and treatment of non-ST-segment elevation acute coronary syndromes: large-scale observations from the CRUSADE (Can Rapid Risk Stratification of Unstable Angina Patients Suppress Adverse Outcomes With Early Implementation of the American College of Cardiology/American Heart Association Guidelines) National Quality Improvement Initiative. J Am Coll Cardiol 2005;45: 832–7.

65. Cotter G, Kaluski E, Milo O, et al. LINCS: L-NAME (a NO synthase inhibitor) in the treatment of refractory cardiogenic shock: a prospective randomized study. Eur Heart J 2003;24:1287–95.

66. Clarke KW, Gray D, Keating NA, et al. Do women with acute myocardial infarction receive the same treatment as men? BMJ 1994;309:563–6.

67. Maynard C, Althouse R, Cerqueira M, et al. Underutilization of thrombolytic therapy in eligible women with acute myocardial infarction. Am J Cardiol 1991;68:529–30.

68. Cariou A, Himbert D, Golmard JL, et al. Sex-related differences in eligibility for reperfusion therapy and in-hospital outcome after acute myocardial infarction. Eur Heart J 1997;18:1583–9.

69. Weaver WD, White HD, Wilcox RG, et al. Comparisons of characteristics and outcomes among

women and men with acute myocardial infarction treated with thrombolytic therapy. GUSTO-I investigators. JAMA 1996;275:777–82.

70. Sanborn TA, Sleeper LA, Bates ER, et al. Impact of thrombolysis, intra-aortic balloon pump counterpulsation, and their combination in cardiogenic shock complicating acute myocardial infarction: a report from the SHOCK Trial Registry. SHould we emergently revascularize Occluded Coronaries for cardiogenic shocK? J Am Coll Cardiol 2000;36:1123–9.

71. Keeley EC, Boura JA, Grines CL. Primary angioplasty versus intravenous thrombolytic therapy for acute myocardial infarction: a quantitative review of 23 randomised trials. Lancet 2003;361:13–20.

72. Hochman JS, Sleeper LA, Webb JG, et al. Early revascularization and long-term survival in cardiogenic shock complicating acute myocardial infarction. JAMA 2006;295:2511–5.

73. Thiele H, Schindler K, Friedenberger J, et al. Intracoronary compared with intravenous bolus abciximab application in patients with ST-elevation myocardial infarction undergoing primary percutaneous coronary intervention: the Randomized Leipzig Immediate Percutaneous Coronary Intervention Abciximab IV Versus IC in ST-Elevation Myocardial Infarction Trial. Circulation 2008;118:49–57.

74. Iversen A, Abildgaard U, Galloe A, et al. Intracoronary compared to intravenous bolus abciximab during primary percutaneous coronary intervention in ST-segment elevation myocardial infarction (STEMI) patients reduces 30-day mortality and target vessel revascularization: a randomized trial. J Interv Cardiol 2011;24:105–11.

75. Gibson CM, Zorkun C, Kunadian V. Intracoronary administration of abciximab in ST-elevation myocardial infarction. Circulation 2008;118:6–8.

76. Kunadian V, Zorkun C, Williams SP, et al. Intracoronary pharmacotherapy in the management of coronary microvascular dysfunction. J Thromb Thrombolysis 2008;26:234–42.

77. Aymong ED, Curtis MJ, Youssef M, et al. Abciximab attenuates coronary microvascular endothelial dysfunction after coronary stenting. Circulation 2002;105:2981–5.

78. Klein LW, Shaw RE, Krone RJ, et al. Mortality after emergent percutaneous coronary intervention in cardiogenic shock secondary to acute myocardial infarction and usefulness of a mortality prediction model. Am J Cardiol 2005;96:35–41.

79. Vijayalakshmi K, Whittaker VJ, Kunadian B, et al. Prospective, randomised, controlled trial to study the effect of intracoronary injection of verapamil and adenosine on coronary blood flow during percutaneous coronary intervention in patients with acute coronary syndromes. Heart 2006;92:1278–84.

80. Stoel MG, Marques KM, de Cock CC, et al. High dose adenosine for suboptimal myocardial reperfusion after primary PCI: a randomized placebo-controlled pilot study. Catheter Cardiovasc Interv 2008;71:283–9.

81. Fokkema ML, Vlaar PJ, Vogelzang M, et al. Effect of high-dose intracoronary adenosine administration during primary percutaneous coronary intervention in acute myocardial infarction: a randomized controlled trial. Circ Cardiovasc Interv 2009;2:323–9.

82. Hussain F. Adenosine conditioning and pacing in conjunction with early intra-aortic balloon pump use and glycoprotein IIb/IIIa inhibition to accomplish complete multivessel revascularization in an octogenarian with profound cardiogenic shock. J Invasive Cardiol 2007;19:E309–12.

83. Perera D, Stables R, Thomas M, et al. Elective intra-aortic balloon counterpulsation during high-risk percutaneous coronary intervention: a randomized controlled trial. JAMA 2010;304:867–74.

84. Patel MR, Smalling RW, Thiele H, et al. Intra-aortic balloon counterpulsation and infarct size in patients with acute anterior myocardial infarction without shock: the CRISP AMI randomized trial. JAMA 2011;306:1329–37.

85. Sjauw KD, Engstrom AE, Vis MM, et al. A systematic review and meta-analysis of intra-aortic balloon pump therapy in ST-elevation myocardial infarction: should we change the guidelines? Eur Heart J 2009;30:459–68.

86. Thiele H, Schuler G. Cardiogenic shock: to pump or not to pump? Eur Heart J 2009;30:389–90.

87. Seyfarth M, Sibbing D, Bauer I, et al. A randomized clinical trial to evaluate the safety and efficacy of a percutaneous left ventricular assist device versus intra-aortic balloon pumping for treatment of cardiogenic shock caused by myocardial infarction. J Am Coll Cardiol 2008;52:1584–8.

88. Cheng JM, den Uil CA, Hoeks SE, et al. Percutaneous left ventricular assist devices vs. intra-aortic balloon pump counterpulsation for treatment of cardiogenic shock: a meta-analysis of controlled trials. Eur Heart J 2009;30:2102–8.

89. Thiele H, Sick P, Boudriot E, et al. Randomized comparison of intra-aortic balloon support with a percutaneous left ventricular assist device in patients with revascularized acute myocardial infarction complicated by cardiogenic shock. Eur Heart J 2005;26:1276–83.

90. Anderson M, Smedira N, Samuels L, et al. Use of the AB5000 ventricular assist device in cardiogenic shock after acute myocardial infarction. Ann Thorac Surg 2010;90:706–12.

91. Shapira I, Isakov A, Burke M, et al. Cardiac rupture in patients with acute myocardial infarction. Chest 1987;92:219–23.

92. Thompson CR, Buller CE, Sleeper LA, et al. Cardio-genic shock due to acute severe mitral regurgitation complicating acute myocardial infarction: a report from the SHOCK Trial Registry. SHould we use emergently revascularize Occluded Coronaries in cardiogenic shocK? J Am Coll Cardiol 2000;36: 1104–9.

93. Menon V, Webb JG, Hillis LD, et al. Outcome and profile of ventricular septal rupture with cardiogenic shock after myocardial infarction: a report from the SHOCK Trial Registry. SHould we emergently revas-cularize Occluded Coronaries in cardiogenic shocK? J Am Coll Cardiol 2000;36:1110–6.

94. Jacobs AK, Leopold JA, Bates E, et al. Cardiogenic shock caused by right ventricular infarction: a report from the SHOCK registry. J Am Coll Cardiol 2003;41: 1273–9.

95. Parodi G, Bellandi B, Del Pace S, et al. Natural history of tako-tsubo cardiomyopathy. Chest 2011; 139:887–92.

# Percutaneous Valve Therapy: Choosing the Appropriate Patients and Outcomes

A. Sonia Petronio, MD*, Cristina Giannini, MD

**KEYWORDS**

- Surgical aortic valve replacement
- Transcatheter aortic valve replacement • Aortic stenosis
- Gender difference

The most frequent native valve disease in industrialized countries today is aortic stenosis (AS), which is most often seen in elderly patients with comorbidities.[1–3] The progressive onset of symptoms such as angina, syncope, and congestive heart failure usually leads to death within 2 to 3 years, unless the patient undergoes surgical aortic valve replacement (SAVR), the current gold standard for the treatment of severe symptomatic AS.[4–6] Operative mortality of SAVR is low, even in elderly patients when properly selected, and long-term results have been shown to be satisfactory.[7,8] However, as the surgical risk is definitely higher in elderly patients when severe comorbidities are present, many patients are not referred for SAVR and are left with a dismal prognosis.[9,10] Transcatheter aortic valve implantation (TAVI) currently represents a viable alternative to conventional SAVR for patients with severe symptomatic AS who are at high risk of operative mortality.[11] Since the first-in-man procedure in 2002, several improvements have been achieved in TAVI device technologies and procedural management, leading to incremental success rates.[12] TAVI has consistently demonstrated good results compared with medical therapy from the pioneering reports to the first randomized trial, showing that this relatively new treatment is safe and effective in inoperable patients and in patients at high risk for surgery. The author's group[13] has recently demonstrated,

in an observational registry study, that in a population of high-risk subjects with several comorbidities, TAVI treatment was associated with lower cardiac mortality with respect to medical management and aortic balloon valvuloplasty. Furthermore, the clinical outcome at 6 months was similar to that in patients undergoing SAVR. In the randomized placement of aortic transcatheter valves (PARTNER) trial, the first multicenter and randomized clinical trial of TAVI, a subgroup of patients with AS who were not candidates for SAVR and who underwent transfemoral placement had an improvement of 20% in the 1-year survival rate and reduced symptoms.[14]

Additional recent evidence has shown that in high-risk patients with severe AS, transcatheter and surgical procedures for aortic valve replacement were associated with similar rates of survival at 1 year (24.2% vs 26.8%, respectively; $P = .62$; noninferiority $P = .001$), although there were important differences in periprocedural risks.[15]

At present, 2 TAVI devices are under postmarketing surveillance in Europe. The first is the Edwards SAPIEN valve (Edwards Lifesciences Inc, Irvine, CA, USA), which consists of 3 pericardial bovine leaflets mounted within a balloon-expandable stent. The other device is the CoreValve Revalving prosthesis (Medtronic Inc, Minneapolis, MN, USA), which has 3 pericardial porcine leaflets mounted in a self-expanding nitinol frame.

Cardiac Catheterization Laboratory, Cardiothoracic and Vascular Department, University of Pisa, via Paradisa n°2, Pisa 46100, Italy
* Corresponding author.
E-mail addresses: as.petronio@gmail.com; spetronio@unipi.it

Intervent Cardiol Clin 1 (2012) 245–250
doi:10.1016/j.iccl.2012.01.005
2211-7458/12/$ – see front matter © 2012 Elsevier Inc. All rights reserved.

interventional.theclinics.com

## GENDER DIFFERENCES IN TREATMENT AND OUTCOME IN SEVERE AS

Several studies have shown gender differences in the treatment and outcomes of ischemic heart disease. These studies indicated that women undergoing coronary artery bypass graft surgery have higher mortality and cardiac morbidity than men.[16–18] In addition, other investigators have identified discrepancies in the rate of use of diagnostic testing and therapy between women and men with known or suspected coronary artery disease.[19,20]

Although gender differences in cardiovascular disease have been explored for a long time, only a limited number of studies have been conducted to show differences between male and female patients with AS, in terms of clinical presentation and outcome after SAVR. Female patients with symptomatic AS tend to be older, more symptomatic, and with more associated advanced disease.[21,22] Despite this, it has been shown that women who underwent SAVR had outcomes similar to those for men.[23] Furthermore, Fuchs and colleagues[24] reported that in patients older than 79 years, women had significantly better survival outcomes after SAVR compared with men. A recent study demonstrated that although women have more late strokes after valve replacement, compared with men they undergo fewer reoperations and have better overall long-term survival.[25] However, despite similar or even better outcomes after surgery, women with severe AS are less likely than men to undergo SAVR.[23–26]

Bach and colleagues[26] have shown that women and patients older than 80 years had lower rates of referral to a specialist, diagnostic testing, and SAVR compared with men and patients aged 65 to 79 years. In particular, SAVR was performed at approximately half the rate in women (1.4%) compared with men (2.7%, P<.001), and in patients older than 80 years (1.1%) compared with those aged 65 to 79 years (2.5%, P<.001).

Lower rates of SAVR in women may have been due to excessive operative risks that would preclude safe intervention. At presentation, female patients with severe AS have a higher predicted operative risk related to the presence of more comorbidities, lower body surface area, and older age.[24] In addition, the EuroScore, which is frequently used for risk assessment of patients undergoing SAVR, calculates an increased risk for women. Recent reports have demonstrated that although female gender may increase the risk for coronary artery bypass surgery, this may not apply to aortic valve replacement.[24]

It has been shown that women receive medical care later than men, either because they wait longer before visiting a doctor or because it takes longer until they are referred to surgery. Women therefore may be more suited to undergo TAVI in view of their coexisting conditions, and may well derive greater benefit.

Several studies have emphasized the existence of sex differences in the left ventricular (LV) adaptation to AS.[22,27] In particular, Carroll and colleagues[22] have observed that women with severe AS are more likely than men to respond to the pressure load with concentric hypertrophy, small volume, and supernormal ejection performance. This finding is in agreement with the preliminary data from the Italian Percutaneous Valve Registry (**Table 1**). The advanced symptomatic status of women has been attributed to more severe LV hypertrophy and, consequently, to more severe LV diastolic function at presentation.

Controversy remains, however, on the impact of sex differences on clinical outcome. The published studies are heterogeneous and with contrasting results.[22,27,28] In some series, this pattern of LV geometry has been associated with increased surgical mortality in women,[28] whereas other series have noted significant differences in LV function and LV geometry among women and men with isolated severe AS, without noting differences in surgical mortality or long-term outcome after SAVR.[27]

Furthermore, on multivariate analysis it has been shown that female gender is independently associated with better recovery of LV systolic function after TAVI[29] and that LV hypertrophy reverses more frequently in female patients after SAVR.[30] During follow-up, however, women remained significantly more symptomatic than men, because at presentation they were significantly older and had more advanced valve disease.[24]

## GENDER DIFFERENCES IN PERCUTANEOUS AORTIC VALVE IMPLANTATION

The available TAVI data show that women are represented more than in previous coronary clinical trials, in which the inclusion rate of female patients has historically been low. In the PARTNER trial, in the subgroup of patients who were not candidates for SAVR and who underwent TAVI, 54.2% of participants were female, whereas in the subgroup of patients at high surgical risk who were assigned to undergo TAVI, 42.2% were female.[14,15] Furthermore, Clavel and colleagues[29] showed that patients treated by TAVI were older and were more frequently women than patients treated by SAVR. Regarding the baseline characteristics of the TAVI population according to sex, women presented with more severe symptoms, smaller body surface area, smaller aortic annulus, and

**Table 1**
**Baseline characteristics of the study population**

|  | Men (n = 483) | Women (n = 585) | P Value |
|---|---|---|---|
| Age (y) | 81.0 ± 7.0 | 83.0 ± 5.0 | <.0001 |
| Logistic EuroScore (%) | 23.9 ± 15.1 | 22.4 ± 13.1 | .05 |
| Annulus MSCT (mm) | 25.0 ± 2.1 | 22.8 ± 2.1 | <.0001 |
| Annulus echo (mm) | 23.5 ± 2.0 | 21.4 ± 1.8 | <.0001 |
| LV outflow tract (mm) | 21.1 ± 2.3 | 19.1 ± 2.2 | <.0001 |
| LVEDD echo (mm) | 53.0 ± 8.0 | 49.7 ± 7.0 | <.0001 |
| LVEDV echo (mm) | 128.0 ± 47.0 | 96.0 ± 33.0 | <.0001 |
| LVEF echo (%) | 49.0 ± 13.1 | 52.8 ± 12.5 | <.0001 |
| IVSTD thickness echo (mm) | 13.4 ± 2.0 | 13.6 ± 2.0 | .17 |
| PWTD thickness echo (mm) | 12.2 ± 2.1 | 12.3 ± 2.1 | .61 |
| LV mass index (g/m$^2$) | 157.0 ± 38.0 | 148.0 ± 38.0 | .002 |
| LV-aortic peak gradient (mm Hg) | 79.0 ± 22.0 | 88.0 ± 26.0 | <.0001 |
| LV-aortic mean gradient (mm Hg) | 48.0 ± 14.0 | 54.0 ± 17.0 | <.0001 |
| EOAi (cm$^2$/m$^2$) | 0.47 ± 0.21 | 0.42 ± 0.22 | .0001 |
| Left femoral artery diameter angio (mm) | 7.9 ± 1.5 | 7.4 ± 1.2 | <.0001 |
| Right femoral artery diameter angio (mm) | 7.8 ± 1.7 | 7.4 ± 1.1 | <.0001 |
| Left femoral artery diameter MSCT (mm) | 8.4 ± 1.6 | 7.6 ± 1.2 | <.0001 |
| Right femoral artery diameter MSCT (mm) | 8.3 ± 1.7 | 7.8 ± 1.4 | .0001 |

Values are means ± SD.

*Abbreviations:* angio, angiography; echo, echocardiography; EOAi, effective aortic valve area index; IVSTD, interventricular septum telediastolic; LV, left ventricular; LVEDD, left ventricular end-systolic diameter; LVEDV, left ventricular end-diastolic volume; LVEF, left ventricular ejection fraction; MSCT, multislice computed tomography; PWTD, posterior wall telediastolic.

more comorbidities compared with their male counterparts.[31] The preliminary data of an ongoing analysis of the Italian Registry are in accordance with these findings (see **Table 1**).

The higher number of women included in TAVI series compared with coronary artery disease series could depend on several factors. The lower body surface area in female patients, which is known to be associated with lower survival after SAVR, could have influenced the therapeutic decision and led to TAVI. Furthermore, it has been noted that the left ventricle of women adapts differently to AS, developing more pronounced hypertrophy with a supernormal ejection fraction, which could have influenced the time of the diagnosis, with symptoms appearing later, thus leading to intervention in women at an older age.[22,32]

To date, few studies have been published regarding gender differences in early and long-term outcomes after TAVI with heterogeneous results.[15,31,33] The PARTNER trial showed a significant interaction for the rate of death at 1 year according to sex, favoring TAVI in women. Women (42.8%) treated with TAVI had a lower mortality at 12 months compared with men (18.4% vs 28.0%). Furthermore, there was a lower 1-year

mortality in women undergoing TAVI compared with SAVR (18.4% vs 27.2%). Similarly, in the French TAVI Registry the 1-year survival estimate was higher for women than for men (76% vs 65%; P = .02), and male gender was a strong and independent predictor of 1-year mortality after TAVI.[34] By contrast, Buchanan and colleagues[31] did not observe significant differences in death rates (3.8% vs 5.6%; P = .47) and cardiovascular death (3.2% vs 4.2%; P = .69) between men and women 30 days after TAVI. In accordance with these results, univariable and multivariable analysis of 1-year mortality in the SOURCE (SAPIEN Aortic Bioprosthesis European Outcome) Registry revealed no differences in the predictors of death according to gender.[33]

Regarding the access site chosen, the available studies are heterogeneous and with contrasting data between sexes.[31,35,36] Buchanan and colleagues[31] found no differences between men and women regarding the access site used (transapical 5.7% vs 8.9%, P = .27; transaxillary 11.9% vs 8.2%, P = .21; transaortic 1.3% vs 0.7%, P = .61). Moreover, in the SOURCE Registry of the Edwards SAPIEN valve, 55.2% of the transfemoral group and 56.0% of the transapical group were female.[35]

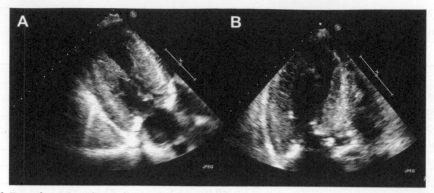

**Fig. 1.** (*A, B*) Transthoracic echocardiographic images of a woman with severe AS, showing asymmetric left ventricular hypertrophy and small left ventricular outflow tract.

In contrast to these studies, the author's group[36] found significant sex differences in a population of 54 patients who underwent TAVI using the subclavian approach (33% women vs 67% men, *P* = .0004), because of the higher prevalence of peripheral artery disease among men.

Several studies have demonstrated the existence of sex differences in the LV adaptation to AS.[22,27] Women had smaller left ventricles with concentric hypertrophy and hyperdynamic LV systolic function. All these baseline characteristics are important in understanding the pathophysiology of AS and have practical consequences for the management and choice of TAVI. TAVI patients are highly prone to complications caused by stiff wire manipulation and possible LV perforation. Asymmetric LV hypertrophy and a small LV outflow tract are frequent among women and need a high, careful valve implantation; the choice of the device can be crucial (**Fig. 1**). Moreover, the smaller annulus size could have a higher risk for aortic dissection or rupture in women than in men. Care needs to be taken when deciding on the most appropriate type and size of percutaneous valve.

It has recently been reported that despite similar rates in device success, female patients receiving TAVI are more likely to have more major vascular complications (19.9% vs 11.9%; *P* = .05) and consequently undergo more blood transfusions than their male counterparts (50.0% vs 38.4%; *P* = .04).[31] Vascular complications in association with the transfemoral approach are not rare and correlate significantly with 30-day mortality.[37] Despite these findings, there was no significant difference in the ileofemoral size between groups (8.9 ± 1.4 mm in women vs 9.8 ± 3.6 mm in men).

## GENDER DIFFERENCES IN THE ITALIAN PERCUTANEOUS AORTIC VALVE REGISTRY

The author analyzed retrospectively 1068 consecutive patients who underwent TAVI from September 2007 to March 2011. Of these, 483 (45.2%) were male and 585 (54.8%) were female. The baseline characteristics of the study population according to sex are summarized in **Table 1**. Mean age and Logistic EuroScore were significantly higher in women than in men (*P*<.0001 and *P*<.05, respectively). Women undergoing TAVI presented higher transvalvular gradients with concomitant smaller valve areas indexed to the body surface area and mean aortic annulus diameter (*P*<.0001). In agreement with previous studies, significant differences in LV function and LV geometry were noted.[27,30] Women had smaller left ventricles with concentric hypertrophy and hyperdynamic LV systolic function. Furthermore, all patients underwent percutaneous angiography and/or multislice computed tomography to evaluate the size, tortuosity, and calcification of peripheral arteries. It was observed that, compared with men, women had a smaller ileofemoral size (*P*<.0001). These findings may explain why female patients are more likely to have major vascular complications, and consequently undergo more blood transfusions than male patients. Buchanan and colleagues[31] have shown that gender is an independent predictor of vascular complications. To date, little is known regarding the gender-specific effects on the outcomes of patients undergoing TAVI.[15,31] In the author's experience, no significant differences between men and women were noted in overall mortality (9.1% vs 7.1%; *P* = .21) and cardiovascular death (7.0% vs 5.6%; *P* = .34) at 30 days.[31] Conversely, a significantly better long-term outcome among women (*P* = .05) was observed.

## SUMMARY

The role of female gender in TAVI is very different from that in other diseases such as coronary artery disease; it is probable that the increase in female life expectancy is a contributory factor in the higher number of female patients scheduled for TAVI. Further investigation of specific gender characteristics in aortic valve disease is warranted with regard to clinical presentation and procedural results, as such factors drive the surgeon's choice and timing of procedures. In the future, more prospective data must be collected, aimed at a full understanding of the differences between male and female patients.

## REFERENCES

1. Iung B, Baron G, Butchart EG, et al. A prospective survey of patients with valvular heart disease in Europe: the Euro Heart Survey on Valvular Heart Disease. Eur Heart J 2003;24(13):1231–43.
2. Carabello BA, Paulus WJ. Aortic stenosis. Lancet 2009;373(9667):956–66.
3. Nkomo VT, Gardin JM, Skelton TN, et al. Burden of valvular heart diseases: a population-based study. Lancet 2006;368(9540):1005–11.
4. Vahanian A, Baumgartner H, Bax J, et al. Guidelines on the management of valvular heart disease: the Task Force on the Management of Valvular Heart Disease of the European Society of Cardiology. Eur Heart J 2007;28(2):230–68.
5. Varadarajan P, Kapoor N, Bansal RC, et al. Clinical profile and natural history of 453 nonsurgically managed patients with severe aortic stenosis. Ann Thorac Surg 2006;82(6):2111–5.
6. Bonow RO, Carabello BA, Chatterjee K, et al. 2008 focused update incorporated into the ACC/AHA 2006 guidelines for the management of patients with valvular heart disease: a report of the American College of Cardiology/American Heart Association Task Force on Practice Guidelines (Writing Committee to Revise the 1998 Guidelines for the Management of Patients With Valvular Heart Disease): endorsed by the Society of Cardiovascular Anesthesiologists, Society for Cardiovascular Angiography and Interventions, and Society of Thoracic Surgeons. Circulation 2008;118(15):e523–661.
7. Kolh P, Lahaye L, Gerard P, et al. Aortic valve replacement in the octogenarians: perioperative outcome and clinical follow-up. Eur J Cardiothorac Surg 1999;16(1):68–73.
8. Sharma UC, Barenbrug P, Pokharel S, et al. Systematic review of the outcome of aortic valve replacement in patients with aortic stenosis. Ann Thorac Surg 2004;78(1):90–5.
9. Chiappini B, Camurri N, Loforte A, et al. Outcome after aortic valve replacement in octogenarians. Ann Thorac Surg 2004;78(1):85–9.
10. Iung B, Cachier A, Baron G, et al. Decision-making in elderly patients with severe aortic stenosis: why are so many denied surgery? Eur Heart J 2005; 26(24):2714–20.
11. Grube E, Laborde JC, Gerckens U, et al. Percutaneous implantation of the CoreValve self-expanding valve prosthesis in high-risk patients with aortic valve disease: the Siegburg first-in-man study. Circulation 2006;114(15):1616–24.
12. Cribier A, Eltchaninoff H, Tron C. First human transcatheter implantation of an aortic valve prosthesis in a case of severe calcific aortic stenosis. Ann Cardiol Angeiol (Paris) 2003;52(3):173–5 [in French].
13. De Carlo M, Giannini C, Ettori F, et al. Impact of treatment choice on the outcome of patients proposed for transcatheter aortic valve implantation. EuroIntervention 2010;6(5):568–74.
14. Leon MB, Smith CR, Mack M, et al. Transcatheter aortic-valve implantation for aortic stenosis in patients who cannot undergo surgery. N Engl J Med 2010;363(17):1597–607.
15. Smith CR, Leon MB, Mack MJ, et al. Transcatheter versus surgical aortic-valve replacement in high-risk patients. N Engl J Med 2011;364(23):2187–98.
16. Guru V, Fremes SE, Austin PC, et al. Gender differences in outcomes after hospital discharge from coronary artery bypass grafting. Circulation 2006; 113(4):507–16.
17. Rankin JS, Hammill BG, Ferguson TB Jr, et al. Determinants of operative mortality in valvular heart surgery. J Thorac Cardiovasc Surg 2006;131(3):547–57.
18. Vaccarino V, Abramson JL, Veledar E, et al. Sex differences in hospital mortality after coronary artery bypass surgery: evidence for a higher mortality in younger women. Circulation 2002;105(10):1176–81.
19. Ayanian JZ, Epstein AM. Differences in the use of procedures between women and men hospitalized for coronary heart disease. N Engl J Med 1991; 325(4):221–5.
20. Roger VL, Farkouh ME, Weston SA, et al. Sex differences in evaluation and outcome of unstable angina. JAMA 2000;283(5):646–52.
21. Duncan AI, Lin J, Koch CG, et al. The impact of gender on in-hospital mortality and morbidity after isolated aortic valve replacement. Anesth Analg 2006;103(4):800–8.
22. Carroll JD, Carroll EP, Feldman T, et al. Sex-associated differences in left ventricular function in aortic stenosis of the elderly. Circulation 1992;86(4):1099–107.
23. Hartzell M, Malhotra R, Yared K, et al. Effect of gender on treatment and outcomes in severe aortic stenosis. Am J Cardiol 2011;107(11):1681–6.
24. Fuchs C, Mascherbauer J, Rosenhek R, et al. Gender differences in clinical presentation and surgical outcome of aortic stenosis. Heart 2010; 96(7):539–45.
25. Kulik A, Lam BK, Rubens FD, et al. Gender differences in the long-term outcomes after valve replacement surgery. Heart 2009;95(4):318–26.
26. Bach DS, Radeva JI, Birnbaum HG, et al. Prevalence, referral patterns, testing, and surgery in aortic

valve disease: leaving women and elderly patients behind? J Heart Valve Dis 2007;16(4):362–9.

27. Milavetz DL, Hayes SN, Weston SA, et al. Sex differences in left ventricular geometry in aortic stenosis: impact on outcome. Chest 2000;117(4):1094–9.

28. Orsinelli DA, Aurigemma GP, Battista S, et al. Left ventricular hypertrophy and mortality after aortic valve replacement for aortic stenosis. A high risk subgroup identified by preoperative relative wall thickness. J Am Coll Cardiol 1993;22(6):1679–83.

29. Clavel MA, Webb JG, Rodes-Cabau J, et al. Comparison between transcatheter and surgical prosthetic valve implantation in patients with severe aortic stenosis and reduced left ventricular ejection fraction. Circulation 2010;122(19):1928–36.

30. Petrov G, Regitz-Zagrosek V, Lehmkuhl E, et al. Regression of myocardial hypertrophy after aortic valve replacement: faster in women? Circulation 2010;122(Suppl 11):S23–8.

31. Buchanan GL, Chieffo A, Montorfano M, et al. The role of sex on VARC outcomes following transcatheter aortic valve implantation with both Edwards SAPIEN and Medtronic CoreValve ReValving System(R) devices: the Milan registry. EuroIntervention 2011;7(5):556–63.

32. Landi F, Onder G, Gambassi G, et al. Body mass index and mortality among hospitalized patients. Arch Intern Med 2000;160(17):2641–4.

33. Thomas M, Schymik G, Walther T, et al. One-year outcomes of cohort 1 in the Edwards SAPIEN Aortic Bioprosthesis European Outcome (SOURCE) registry: the European Registry of Transcatheter Aortic Valve Implantation using the Edwards SAPIEN valve. Circulation 2011;124(4):425–33.

34. European Society of Cardiology. Gender differences in clinical presentation and outcome of transcatheter aortic valve implantation (TAVI) for severe aortic stenosis. Press release from ESC Congress 2011. Paris, August 29, 2011.

35. Thomas M, Schymik G, Walther T, et al. Thirty-day results of the SAPIEN aortic Bioprosthesis European Outcome (SOURCE) Registry: A European registry of transcatheter aortic valve implantation using the Edwards SAPIEN valve. Circulation 2010;122(1): 62–9.

36. Petronio AS, De Carlo M, Bedogni F, et al. Safety and efficacy of the subclavian approach for transcatheter aortic valve implantation with the CoreValve revalving system. Circ Cardiovasc Interv 2010;3(4):359–66.

37. Piazza N, Grube E, Gerckens U, et al. Procedural and 30-day outcomes following transcatheter aortic valve implantation using the third generation (18 Fr) CoreValve revalving system: results from the multicentre, expanded evaluation registry 1-year following CE mark approval. EuroIntervention 2008; 4(2):242–9.

# Future Perspectives on Percutaneous Coronary Interventions in Women

Jennifer Conroy, MD, MBE*, Usman Baber, MD, MS, Roxana Mehran, MD

## KEYWORDS

• Percutaneous coronary interventions • PCI • Women
• Coronary disease • Future perspectives

It has been more than 3 decades since Dr Andreas Gruentzig performed the first percutaneous angioplasty in a human coronary artery. There have been dramatic advances in interventional cardiology since that first successful percutaneous coronary intervention (PCI). In the United States alone, more than a million cardiac catheterizations are performed each year, with approximately 600,000 patients undergoing PCI.[1]

A meaningful perspective on the future of PCI in women requires not only reflection on some of the major developments in interventional cardiology but also a look back more generally at the changing patterns in the burden of coronary disease in the population and at the gains accrued in understanding and combating cardiovascular disease (CVD) in women. Developments in revascularization strategies, evolving stent technology, management of procedural complications, and the creation of scoring models for risk stratification have dramatically changed PCI for all patients. For women in particular, these developments lay the foundation for a future that holds great promise in the use of PCI for the management of coronary disease. However, there have often been conflicting findings with respect to the validity and applicability of these advances to the clinical management of women with coronary disease. These concerns identify areas ripe for future research. Identifying major barriers in the management of women with coronary disease is critical for ensuring that future generations of women benefit from advances in PCI. Improving education on the burden of coronary disease in women and increasing representation of women in major clinical trials are essential to uncovering answers to recurring questions on the impact of gender on outcomes in PCI.

## EPIDEMIOLOGY OF CVD

With the exception of 1918, CVD has been the leading cause of death for both men and women in the United States since 1900. However, the mortality associated with CVD has declined significantly over time. Most recently, between 1997 and 2007 the mortality for CVD decreased by nearly 28%. Mortality for coronary heart disease (CHD) has similarly declined for the general population, decreasing by nearly 27% between the years 1997 and 2007.[1]

What accounts for the decrease in mortality for CHD? In addition to increased public awareness, major advances in medical therapies and coronary revascularization have fueled these gains. In concert with evolving medical therapies, the advent of thrombolytic therapy followed by the development and refinement of PCI has significantly affected the morbidity and mortality for CHD.

However, despite these improvements, CVD remains the leading cause of death in the United States and accounts for 1 in every 3 deaths in the general population according to most recent statistics. In women, the number of deaths attributable to CVD exceeded that caused by cancer, chronic lung disease, and Alzheimer disease combined (**Fig. 1**). Since 1984, the yearly absolute

Department of Medicine, Mount Sinai School of Medicine, One Gustave L. Levy Place, Box 1030, New York, NY 10029, USA
* Corresponding author.
E-mail address: Jennifer.conroy@mountsinai.org

Intervent Cardiol Clin 1 (2012) 251–258
doi:10.1016/j.iccl.2012.02.003

interventional.theclinics.com

number of CVD-related deaths for women has been higher than those in men.[1]

CHD, specifically, accounted for nearly 1 in every 6 deaths in the United States in 2007.[1,2] In women, CHD accounted for nearly half of all CVD deaths.[3,4] Of additional concern, in young women (35–44 years of age), as opposed to every other age and gender group, mortality related to CHD increased approximately 1.3% per year between 1997 and 2002.[1,3,5] It is clear from these statistics that significant progress is needed in the battle against heart disease in women.

## REVASCULARIZATION STRATEGIES

Although there is currently an appreciation of the burden of disease in women, coronary disease was historically considered an illness of men. Throughout the 1950s and 1960s, information available in scientific, professional, and lay publications on coronary disease focused on a woman's role in preventing "heart disease in husbands and helping husbands after a heart attack." In the 1970s, the presence of coronary disease in women was attributed to lifestyle factors such as smoking, the use of oral contraception, and the increasing trend of women entering the national work force.[6]

However, there is greater general knowledge not only with respect to the occurrence of disease in women but also about the distinct patterns and presentation of CHD in women. For example, the overall incidence of CHD is lower in women than in men, except in very elderly individuals. Women are also less likely to have classic angina and more likely to have atypical complaints. Women are on average 10 years older than men at the time of presentation, have more risk factors for coronary disease, higher rates of heart failure, and a greater degree of symptoms, with a similar degree of epicardial disease.[7,8]

Significant disparities remain also in the management of CHD in women. Despite accounting for 40% of the population of Americans with CHD, women account for only one-third of the population undergoing PCI.[1] Women are generally treated less aggressively for acute coronary syndrome (ACS) than men after presentation. In ACS, women are more likely to have increased levels of brain natriuretic peptide and C-reactive protein, whereas men more commonly have increased cardiac markers, including troponin and creatinine kinase-MB. The presence of increased markers is correlated with mortality benefit from early revascularization for both men and women. However, only in women is the absence of positive markers correlated with higher rates of adverse events when undergoing early invasive therapy compared with conservative management.[9–11] Women are less likely to receive reperfusion therapy for ST-elevation myocardial infarction (STEMI), be it with fibrinolytics or primary PCI for STEMI.[12–14] In the hospital, they are less likely to receive treatment with aspirin and statins.[13,15]

A widely held belief has been that women fare more poorly than men undergoing primary PCI for ACS and this belief has been suggested to be the culprit cause for underreferral and observed bias treatment.[15] As early as 1985, an analysis of national registry data revealed that women undergoing angioplasty had lower procedural success rates combined with higher procedural and in-hospital mortality.[16] Contemporary data from CADILLAC (Controlled Abciximab and Device Investigation to Lower Late Angioplasty Complication), a large prospective multicenter randomized clinical trial on reperfusion strategies for acute myocardial infarction (AMI), found that women had higher rates of major adverse cardiac events (MACE), death, and target vessel revascularization at 1 year after intervention. However, statistical analysis revealed that gender did not independently predict mortality at 1 year although it did predict higher rates of MACE and bleeding complications. Importantly, in women, primary PCI for

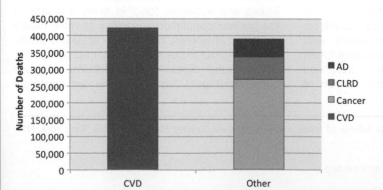

Fig. 1. Leading causes of death in women, 2007. CVD, deaths attributable to total CVD (including deaths attributable to stroke); AD, Alzheimer disease; CLRD, chronic lower respiratory disease. (Data from Roger VL, Go AS, Lloyd-Jones DM, et al. Heart disease and stroke statistics–2011 update: a report from the American Heart Association. Circulation 2011;123(4):e18–209.)

AMI reduced 1-year MACE and ischemic target vessel revascularization compared with angioplasty.[17] In the case of non-STEMI/unstable angina a conservative strategy is given a class I indication, within 2007 American College of Cardiology (ACCF)/American Heart Association (AHA) guidelines for the management of women presenting with low-risk features.[11,18] Recent ACCF/AHA/Society for Cardiovascular Angiography and Interventions (SCAI) guidelines for PCI management of patients with STEMI recognize that women with STEMI are more likely to have worse outcomes compared with men.[19,20] The advent of sex-specific treatment recommendations and discussion of unique care issues within professional guidelines is important for the adoption of standard practice in the management of ACS in women. Looking to the future, elimination of the disparities in referral and treatment of ACS and the further analysis of the differential outcomes for women undergoing PCI are priorities.

## CORONARY STENTING IN WOMEN

The US Food and Drug Administration approved the first intracoronary stent for clinical use in 1994. Early on, concern was raised that success rates for stenting in women were lower, with higher incidences of periprocedural non-STEMI and vascular complications. However, no difference was seen in survival, late myocardial infarction, or repeat revascularization using the first-generation bare-metal Palmaz-Schatz stent.[21] Since then, there has been a dramatic explosion in the types of stents available and in the various stages of research and development. Drug-eluting stents (DES) now account for approximately 80% of stents implanted during PCI.[1] Multiple studies have analyzed the impact of particular DES on outcomes. In the case of sirolimus-eluting and paclitaxel-eluting stents, both seemed to have comparable results in men and women with respect to major adverse cardiac events, reducing restenosis and revascularization rates.[15,22,23] Data from the SPIRIT III (Clinical Evaluation of the Xience V Everolimus Eluting Coronary Stent System in the Treatment of Patients with De Novo Coronary Artery Lesions) trial, a randomized multicenter clinical trial comparing XIENCE V (Abott, Abbott Park, IL, USA) with TAXUS Express2 (paclitaxel-eluting) stents (Boston Scientific, Galway, Ireland) revealed higher rates of MACE, target vessel failure, target vessel revascularization, and target lesion revascularization in women than in men at 1-year follow-up.[24] In the same population, a post hoc gender subset analysis of outcomes at 3 years after intervention concluded that women, overall, had higher rates of major adverse cardiovascular events and target lesion revascularization rates. Women who received XIENCE V stents had lower MACE and similar target vessel failure rates compared with those who received TAXUS.[25] A recent large single-center retrospective analysis of PCI, using multiple stent types, concluded that gender does not predict higher mortality after intervention even at long-term 3-year follow-up.[26] Results from the multicenter XIENCE V SPIRIT Women study, a multicenter prospective open-label, single-arm trial evaluating the use of everolimus-eluting stents in women, may add to our understanding of gender-specific outcomes after DES placement.

Stent thrombosis and restenosis continue to affect the success of DES in both women and men. Future innovations including drug-coated balloons, polymer free DES, biodegradable stents, and novel coatings are being developed, with the goal of reducing this complication.[27,28] Women may particularly benefit from these emerging technologies given the evidence of unadjusted worse outcomes with current stents and the observation of altered endothelial function and higher degrees of small vessel disease, microvascular abnormalities, and arterial vasospasm.[7,8] Clinical trials using these next-generation technologies should strive to enroll adequate numbers of women so that these potential benefits can be appropriately examined.

## BLEEDING AND VASCULAR COMPLICATIONS

Although the data on gender-based outcomes after PCI may often seem conflicting, a preponderance of data have identified increased rates of bleeding and vascular complications for women undergoing PCI than for men.[29,30] Moreover, major bleeding complications have been associated with increased mortality in ACS and PCI.[29,31,32]

The use of glycoprotein IIb/IIIa inhibitors and direct thrombin inhibitors raised concerns of increased vascular complications with these agents in women undergoing PCI. However, results from several large trials did not identify gender as an independent predictor for increased vascular complication with the use of glycoprotein IIb/IIIa inhibitors.[17] From the ACUITY (Acute Catheterization and Urgent Intervention Triage Strategy) trial, a prospective, multicenter, randomized clinical trial, post hoc subgroup analysis revealed that women treated with bivalirudin alone had significantly decreased bleeding rates, compared with those treated with heparin plus glycoprotein IIb/IIIa inhibitor, and maintained similar outcomes with respect to ischemic events both short-term and long-term.[33,34]

The deleterious impact of bleeding on outcomes has spurred the development of risk scores to calculate bleeding risk in a composite group of patients undergoing PCI. Most recently, a risk score was created using pooled analysis from 3 large, randomized clinical trials. Seven variables were identified (of which gender was one) that predict TIMI (Thrombolysis in Myocardial Infarction) major bleeding within 30 days of PCI (**Box 1**). Noncoronary artery bypass graft-related bleeding within 30 days of PCI correlated with increased mortality at 1 year.[35]

Concerns over bleeding and vascular complications have spurred the refinement of access techniques and equipment. Radial access is increasingly used to mitigate these complications. In a registry analysis, the reduction in bleeding complications is more pronounced in women than in men, although the rate of radial catheterization is lower in women than in men.[36] Increasing use of minimally invasive access techniques may help reduce bleeding complications moving forward.

Although studies to date shed new light on outcomes with respect to bleeding complications in women, compared with men, the driving factors for these observed differences remain to be elucidated. It is likely that a combination of factors, including different biologic responses to therapies and differing rates of disease progression, are at play. Future study is required to clearly identify these factors and their causal relationships with observed outcomes in women undergoing PCI.

---

**Box 1**
**Variables that independently predict TIMI major bleeding within 30 days of PCI**

Advanced age

Female gender

White blood cell count

Increased serum creatinine

Abnormal biomarkers

Cigarette smoking

Antithrombotic medications

*Data from* Mehran R, Pocock S, Nikolsky E, et al. Impact of bleeding on mortality after percutaneous coronary intervention results from a patient-level pooled analysis of the REPLACE-2 (randomized evaluation of PCI linking angiomax to reduced clinical events), ACUITY (acute catheterization and urgent intervention triage strategy), and HORIZONS-AMI (harmonizing outcomes with revascularization and stents in acute myocardial infarction) trials. JACC Cardiovasc Interv 2011;4(6):654–64.

---

## CLINICAL RISK SCORES AND WOMEN

Assessing an individual patient's risk before intervention is essential to selecting appropriate plans of care and treatment. The development of risk scores and models in cardiology has affected how patients are treated in the various subspecialties. In interventional cardiology, numerous risk scores exist that predict a variety of outcomes, including angiographic success, MACE, procedural complications (such as bleeding and renal dysfunction), and aid in selecting an appropriate revascularization strategy. For example, the SYNTAX (Synergy between PCI with TAXUS drug-eluting stent and Cardiac Surgery) score was developed as an anatomically derived score quantifying coronary disease severity. Multiple trials have shown that the highest SYNTAX scores correlate with the worst outcomes with respect to PCI. There have been multiple analyses of the SYNTAX score validating its use in risk stratification. Additional refinements with clinical data (Clinical SYNTAX) or alternatively with functional data derived from fractional flow reserve (Functional SYNTAX) enhance the ability of the score to predict outcomes.[37–40] Additional risk models routinely used by interventional cardiologists predicting cardiac operative mortality include the STS (Society of Thoracic Surgeons) score and euroSCORE (European System for Cardiac Operative Risk Evaluation). Although the use of these risk scores has changed the decision-making approach to the care of complex patients, less is known about the accuracy of such scores in women, particularly with the revised scores incorporating clinical and functional data.[41,42] Current models will be refined and new models developed to predict risk. However, as with all studies, women should be adequately represented in the development and validation of these risk scores.

## BARRIERS

Women should continue to benefit from the evolution in revascularization strategies, advances in stent technology, and the reduction in procedural complications. However, there are considerable obstacles related to women's representation in research trials, women's awareness of disease risk, physician's awareness of women's disease risk, and shifting population demographics, which limit the impact these advances may have for women with CHD and merit special attention.

The underrepresentation of women in clinical trials limits the generalizability of findings and guidelines to women as a patient group. An analysis of the 2007 AHA guidelines for CVD disease prevention in women found that representation of women in clinical trials remains suboptimal. Although the percentage of women enrolled in trials referenced in the guidelines increased from 9% in 1970 it remained low at 41% in 2006. Representation was lowest in trials focusing on CHD: women accounted for only 25% of the total population in the studies on CHD. Women were better represented in international trials than in those based only in the United States. Overall, women accounted for less than one-third of the study population in the trials on which the guidelines were based.[43] Several major trials referenced in this article similarly suffer from underrepresentation of women (**Table 1**).

Despite major public awareness campaigns, significant gaps in women's knowledge on their risk for CVD and evidence-based preventative health and risk factor modification remain. In a survey of more than 1000 women in 2009, just 54% of the group was able to correctly identify CVD as the leading cause of death among women. Although this finding represents significant improvement since 1997 (when only 30% of women correctly identified CVD as the major killer of women), there was no significant difference in awareness since 2006. Perhaps of greater concern, only 53% of the women indicated that they would contact emergency services if they felt that they were suffering from an AMI and only 23% reported that they would take an aspirin. There were significant differences in awareness among different racial and ethnic groups, with African American, Hispanic, and Asian women being less likely than white women to be aware of CVD as the leading cause of death.[44]

Physicians may also lack insight into the real risk that women face with respect to CVD. In a survey of 500 practicing physicians, including primary care physicians, obstetricians/gynecologists and cardiologists, less than 20% knew that CVD causes more deaths in women than in men. Only 17% of the 100 surveyed cardiologists were aware of this fact.[45]

These gaps of knowledge are even more concerning when framed in the context of historical and forecasted population trends. Nearly two-thirds of women in the United States are overweight or obese. Obesity in children has nearly tripled since 1980; 17% of youth aged 2 to 19 years are obese. Nearly 11% of women in the United States older than 20 years (12.6 million individuals) have diabetes.[1] Although projections vary, the Centers for Disease Control estimate that the prevalence of diabetes will increase from 8.3% of the general population in 2010 to 21% to 33% in 2050.[46] The elderly population is expected to double by 2050. These projections suggest that left unchecked the current observed disparities in CVD outcomes in women may be magnified by the increasing prevalence of elderly, obese, and diabetic patients. As the prevalence of CVD increases so too will the costs. CVD accounts for 17% of the national health costs; by 2030 the direct costs are expected to triple, whereas indirect costs are expected to increase by 61%. The costs associated with CHD alone are projected to increase by 53%.[47]

These issues have helped to spur the development of global initiatives, women-specific clinical trials, public awareness campaigns, and the creation of women's health and cardiovascular centers in local communities. For example, the Women in Innovations (WIN) initiative, launched by the SCAI, which was created with the mission to "encourage and facilitate more effective diagnosis of and treatment of women with cardiovascular disease," has made inroads in disseminating knowledge of these gender disparities in cardiology.[15]

## SUMMARY

In women, evolution in the use of PCI for the management of CHD has been informed both by insights into shared commonalities of the disease process with men and more recently by new appreciation for unique pathophysiologic processes and responses to interventions and therapeutics. As innovations in pharmacology, technology, and technique continue to shape the promising future of PCI, we must be vigilant that all patients, but particularly women, are beneficiaries of these advances, while at the same time

**Table 1**
**Representation of women in referenced trials**

| Study Patient Population from Which Gender-Based Analyses Performed | Percentage of Women of Study Population |
| --- | --- |
| BARI[7] | 27 |
| TACTIS-TIMI 18[9] | 34 |
| CADILLAC[15] | 27 |
| TAXUS-IV[18] | 28 |
| SPIRIT III[20,21] | 31 |
| GRACE[25] | 23 |
| CRUSADE[26] | 37 |
| ACUITY[28,29] | 30 |
| ESPIRIT[30] | 27 |
| SYNTAX[40] | 22 |

improve education and access for the basic management of CHD.

## REFERENCES

1. Roger VL, Go AS, Lloyd-Jones DM, et al. Heart disease and stroke statistics–2011 update: a report from the American Heart Association. Circulation 2011;123(4):e18–209.

2. Heron M, Hoyert DL, Murphy SL, et al. Deaths: final data for 2006. Natl Vital Stat Rep 2009;57(14):1–134.

3. Mosca L, Benjamin EJ, Berra K, et al. Effectiveness-based guidelines for the prevention of cardiovascular disease in women–2011 update: a guideline from the American Heart Association. J Am Coll Cardiol 2011; 57(12):1404–23.

4. Ford ES, Ajani UA, Croft JB, et al. Explaining the decrease in U.S. deaths from coronary disease, 1980-2000. N Engl J Med 2007;356(23):2388–98.

5. Roger VL, Go AS, Lloyd-Jones DM, et al. Heart disease and stroke statistics–2012 update: a report from the American Heart Association. Circulation 2012;125(1):e2–220.

6. Miller CL, Kollauf CR. Evolution of information on women and heart disease 1957-2000: a review of archival records and secular literature. Heart Lung 2002;31(4):253–61.

7. Jacobs AK, Kelsey SF, Brooks MM, et al. Better outcome for women compared with men undergoing coronary revascularization: a report from the bypass angioplasty revascularization investigation (BARI). Circulation 1998;98(13):1279–85.

8. Davis KB, Chaitman B, Ryan T, et al. Comparison of 15-year survival for men and women after initial medical or surgical treatment for coronary artery disease: a CASS registry study. Coronary Artery Surgery Study. J Am Coll Cardiol 1995;25(5): 1000–9.

9. Wiviott SD, Cannon CP, Morrow DA, et al. Differential expression of cardiac biomarkers by gender in patients with unstable angina/non-ST-elevation myocardial infarction: a TACTICS-TIMI 18 (Treat Angina with Aggrastat and determine Cost of Therapy with an Invasive or Conservative Strategy-Thrombolysis In Myocardial Infarction 18) substudy. Circulation 2004;109(5):580–6.

10. Glaser R, Herrmann HC, Murphy SA, et al. Benefit of an early invasive management strategy in women with acute coronary syndromes. JAMA 2002; 288(24):3124–9.

11. Anderson JL, Adams CD, Antman EM, et al. ACC/AHA 2007 guidelines for the management of patients with unstable angina/non ST-elevation myocardial infarction: a report of the American College of Cardiology/American Heart Association Task Force on Practice Guidelines (Writing Committee to Revise the 2002 Guidelines for the Management of Patients With Unstable Angina/Non

ST-Elevation Myocardial Infarction): developed in collaboration with the American College of Emergency Physicians, the Society for Cardiovascular Angiography and Interventions, and the Society of Thoracic Surgeons: endorsed by the American Association of Cardiovascular and Pulmonary Rehabilitation and the Society for Academic Emergency Medicine. Circulation 2007; 116(7):e148–304.

12. Levine GN, Bates ER, Blankenship JC, et al. 2011 ACCF/AHA/SCAI Guideline for Percutaneous Coronary Intervention. A report of the American College of Cardiology Foundation/American Heart Association Task Force on Practice Guidelines and the Society for Cardiovascular Angiography and Interventions. J Am Coll Cardiol 2011;58(24):e44–122.

13. Jneid H, Fonarow GC, Cannon CP, et al. Sex differences in medical care and early death after acute myocardial infarction. Circulation 2008;118(25): 2803–10.

14. Mehta RH, Bufalino VJ, Pan W, et al. Achieving rapid reperfusion with primary percutaneous coronary intervention remains a challenge: insights from American Heart Association's Get With the Guidelines program. Am Heart J 2008;155(6):1059–67.

15. Chieffo A, Hoye A, Mauri F, et al. Gender-based issues in interventional cardiology: a consensus statement from the Women in Innovations (WIN) Initiative. Catheter Cardiovasc Interv 2010;75(2): 145–52.

16. Cowley MJ, Mullin SM, Kelsey SF, et al. Sex differences in early and long-term results of coronary angioplasty in the NHLBI PTCA Registry. Circulation 1985;71(1):90–7.

17. Lansky AJ, Pietras C, Costa RA, et al. Gender differences in outcomes after primary angioplasty versus primary stenting with and without abciximab for acute myocardial infarction: results of the Controlled Abciximab and Device Investigation to Lower Late Angioplasty Complications (CADILLAC) trial. Circulation 2005;111(13):1611–8.

18. Wright RS, Anderson JL, Adams CD, et al. 2011 ACCF/AHA focused update of the Guidelines for the Management of Patients with Unstable Angina/Non-ST-Elevation Myocardial Infarction (updating the 2007 guideline): a report of the American College of Cardiology Foundation/American Heart Association Task Force on Practice Guidelines developed in collaboration with the American College of Emergency Physicians, Society for Cardiovascular Angiography and Interventions, and Society of Thoracic Surgeons. J Am Coll Cardiol 2011;57(19):1920–59.

19. Levine GN, Bates ER, Blankenship JC, et al. 2011 ACCF/AHA/SCAI Guideline for Percutaneous Coronary Intervention: a report of the American College of Cardiology Foundation/American Heart Association Task Force on Practice Guidelines and the

Society for Cardiovascular Angiography and Interventions. Circulation 2011;124(23):e574–651.

20. Kushner FG, Hand M, Smith SC Jr, et al. 2009 focused updates: ACC/AHA guidelines for the management of patients with ST-elevation myocardial infarction (updating the 2004 guideline and 2007 focused update) and ACC/AHA/SCAI guidelines on percutaneous coronary intervention (updating the 2005 guideline and 2007 focused update) a report of the American College of Cardiology Foundation/American Heart Association Task Force on Practice Guidelines. J Am Coll Cardiol 2009; 54(23):2205–41.

21. Fishman RF, Kuntz RE, Carrozza JP Jr, et al. Acute and long-term results of coronary stents and atherectomy in women and the elderly. Coron Artery Dis 1995;6(2):159–68.

22. Lansky AJ, Costa RA, Mooney M, et al. Gender-based outcomes after paclitaxel-eluting stent implantation in patients with coronary artery disease. J Am Coll Cardiol 2005;45(8):1180–5.

23. Solinas E, Nikolsky E, Lansky AJ, et al. Gender-specific outcomes after sirolimus-eluting stent implantation. J Am Coll Cardiol 2007;50(22): 2111–6.

24. Lansky AJ, Ng VG, Mutlu H, et al. Gender-based evaluation of the XIENCE V everolimus-eluting coronary stent system: clinical and angiographic results from the SPIRIT III randomized trial. Catheter Cardiovasc Interv 2009;74(5):719–27.

25. Ng VG, Lansky AJ, Hermiller JB, et al. Three-year results of safety and efficacy of the everolimus-eluting coronary stent in women (from the SPIRIT III randomized clinical trial). Am J Cardiol 2011; 107(6):841–8.

26. Kovacic JC, Mehran R, Karajgikar R, et al. Female gender and mortality after percutaneous coronary intervention: results from a large registry. Catheter Cardiovasc Interv 2011. [Epub ahead of print].

27. Garg S, Serruys PW. Coronary stents: looking forward. J Am Coll Cardiol 2010;56(Suppl 10):S43–78.

28. Sharma S, Kukreja N, Christopoulos C, et al. Drug-eluting balloon: new tool in the box. Expert Rev Med Devices 2010;7(3):381–8.

29. Moscucci M, Fox KA, Cannon CP, et al. Predictors of major bleeding in acute coronary syndromes: the Global Registry of Acute Coronary Events (GRACE). Eur Heart J 2003;24(20):1815–23.

30. Alexander KP, Chen AY, Newby LK, et al. Sex differences in major bleeding with glycoprotein IIb/IIIa inhibitors: results from the CRUSADE (Can Rapid risk stratification of Unstable angina patients Suppress ADverse outcomes with Early implementation of the ACC/AHA guidelines) initiative. Circulation 2006;114(13):1380–7.

31. Doyle BJ, Rihal CS, Gastineau DA, et al. Bleeding, blood transfusion, and increased mortality after percutaneous coronary intervention: implications for contemporary practice. J Am Coll Cardiol 2009; 53(22):2019–27.

32. Manoukian SV, Feit F, Mehran R, et al. Impact of major bleeding on 30-day mortality and clinical outcomes in patients with acute coronary syndromes: an analysis from the ACUITY Trial. J Am Coll Cardiol 2007;49(12):1362–8.

33. Lansky AJ, Mehran R, Cristea E, et al. Impact of gender and antithrombin strategy on early and late clinical outcomes in patients with non-ST-elevation acute coronary syndromes (from the ACUITY trial). Am J Cardiol 2009;103(9):1196–203.

34. Fernandes LS, Tcheng JE, O'Shea JC, et al. Is glycoprotein IIb/IIIa antagonism as effective in women as in men following percutaneous coronary intervention?. Lessons from the ESPRIT study. J Am Coll Cardiol 2002;40(6):1085–91.

35. Mehran R, Pocock S, Nikolsky E, et al. Impact of bleeding on mortality after percutaneous coronary intervention results from a patient-level pooled analysis of the REPLACE-2 (randomized evaluation of PCI linking angiomax to reduced clinical events), ACUITY (acute catheterization and urgent intervention triage strategy), and HORIZONS-AMI (harmonizing outcomes with revascularization and stents in acute myocardial infarction) trials. JACC Cardiovasc Interv 2011;4(6):654–64.

36. Rao SV, Ou FS, Wang TY, et al. Trends in the prevalence and outcomes of radial and femoral approaches to percutaneous coronary intervention: a report from the National Cardiovascular Data Registry. JACC Cardiovasc Interv 2008;1(4):379–86.

37. Farooq V, Brugaletta S, Serruys PW. Contemporary and evolving risk scoring algorithms for percutaneous coronary intervention. Heart 2011;97(23): 1902–13.

38. Farooq V, Brugaletta S, Serruys PW. Utilizing risk scores in determining the optimal revascularization strategy for complex coronary artery disease. Curr Cardiol Rep 2011;13(5):415–23.

39. Nam CW, Mangiacapra F, Entjes R, et al. Functional SYNTAX score for risk assessment in multivessel coronary artery disease. J Am Coll Cardiol 2011; 58(12):1211–8.

40. Serruys PW, Morice MC, Kappetein AP, et al. Percutaneous coronary intervention versus coronary-artery bypass grafting for severe coronary artery disease. N Engl J Med 2009;360(10):961–72.

41. Ad N, Barnett SD, Speir AM. The performance of the EuroSCORE and the Society of Thoracic Surgeons mortality risk score: the gender factor. Interact Cardiovasc Thorac Surg 2007;6(2):192–5.

42. Massoudy P, Sander J, Wendt D, et al. Does the euroSCORE equally well predict perioperative cardiac surgical risk for men and women? Minim Invasive Ther Allied Technol 2011;20(2):67–71.

43. Melloni C, Berger JS, Wang TY, et al. Representation of women in randomized clinical trials of cardiovascular disease prevention. Circ Cardiovasc Qual Outcomes 2010;3(2):135–42.

44. Mosca L, Mochari-Greenberger H, Dolor RJ, et al. Twelve-year follow-up of American women's awareness of cardiovascular disease risk and barriers to heart health. Circ Cardiovasc Qual Outcomes 2010;3(2):120–7.

45. Mosca L, Linfante AH, Benjamin EJ, et al. National study of physician awareness and adherence to cardiovascular disease prevention guidelines. Circulation 2005;111(4):499–510.

46. Boyle JP, Thompson TJ, Gregg EW, et al. Projection of the year 2050 burden of diabetes in the US adult population: dynamic modeling of incidence, mortality, and prediabetes prevalence. Popul Health Metr 2010;8:29.

47. Heidenreich PA, Trogdon JG, Khavjou OA, et al. Forecasting the future of cardiovascular disease in the United States: a policy statement from the American Heart Association. Circulation 2011;123(8):933–44.

# Index

*Note:* Page numbers of article titles are in **boldface** type.

Intervent Cardiol Clin 1 (2012) 259–263
doi:10.1016/S2211-7458(12)00052-1
2211-7458/12/$ – see front matter © 2012 Elsevier Inc. All rights reserved.

interventional.theclinics.com

# Moving?

## Make sure your subscription moves with you!

To notify us of your new address, find your **Clinics Account Number** (located on your mailing label above your name), and contact customer service at:

**Email: journalscustomerservice-usa@elsevier.com**

**800-654-2452** (subscribers in the U.S. & Canada)
**314-447-8871** (subscribers outside of the U.S. & Canada)

**Fax number: 314-447-8029**

**Elsevier Health Sciences Division**
**Subscription Customer Service**
**3251 Riverport Lane**
**Maryland Heights, MO 63043**

*To ensure uninterrupted delivery of your subscription, please notify us at least 4 weeks in advance of move.

# Moving?

## Make sure your subscription moves with you!

To notify us of your new address, find your Clinics Account Number (located on your mailing label above your name), and contact customer service at:

**Email: journalscustomerservice-usa@elsevier.com**

**800-654-2452** (subscribers in the U.S. & Canada)
**314-447-8871** (subscribers outside of the U.S. & Canada)

Fax number: 314-447-8029

**Elsevier Health Sciences Division**
**Subscription Customer Service**
**3251 Riverport Lane**
**Maryland Heights, MO 63043**

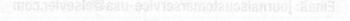
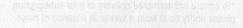

Printed and bound by CPI Group (UK) Ltd, Croydon, CR0 4YY
04/05/2023
01040982-0004

Printed and bound by CPI Group (UK) Ltd, Croydon, CR0 4YY

03/10/2024

01040352-0004